I0094374

Weight Loss Plan For Menopause

Use Your Diet To Get Through Menopause With A 7-Day Weight Loss Plan For Women Suffering From Menopause To Lose Weight and Burn Belly Fat

Yara Green

Dawn Publishing House

© Copyright 2022 - All rights reserved.

The content contained within this book may not be reproduced, duplicated or transmitted without direct written permission from the author or the publisher.

Under no circumstances will any blame or legal responsibility be held against the publisher, or author, for any damages, reparation, or monetary loss due to the information contained within this book, either directly or indirectly.

Legal Notice:

This book is copyright protected. It is only for personal use. You cannot amend, distribute, sell, use, quote or paraphrase any part, or the content within this book, without the consent of the author or publisher.

Disclaimer Notice:

Please note the information contained within this document is for educational and entertainment purposes only. All effort has been executed to present accurate, up to date, reliable, complete information. No warranties of any kind are declared or implied. Readers acknowledge that the author is not engaged in the rendering of legal, financial, medical or professional advice. The content within this book has been derived from various sources. Please consult a licensed professional before attempting any techniques outlined in this book.

By reading this document, the reader agrees that under no circumstances is the author responsible for any losses, direct or indirect, that are incurred as a result of the use of the information contained within this document, including, but not limited to, errors, omissions, or inaccuracies.

Table of Contents

Introduction

Menopause is unpredictable. All women know it is going to come but it hits them suddenly; the hot flashes, the sleepless nights, mood swings they can't explain, and it feels as though they've gained 15 pounds overnight. As natural as it is, menopause can make the most confident women feel unsure about what is going on with them. The hormone changes and the shift in the way your body is storing fat can make you feel like you have let yourself go. It can make you feel like there is nothing you can do about what is going on with your body.

The most common way women used to get through menopause was with hormone treatment. While this option is ideal for many and can help relieve hot flashes and night sweats, it also comes with significant risk. Hormone therapy puts women at greater risk for stroke, heart disease, and even breast cancer. It also does not do much to help with weight gain. But, there is another way!

Understanding what causes most women to gain weight just before and through menopause can help you use the right tools to manage your weight and other changes. Knowing what to expect is the first step. Learning what to do about these changes is the next. You don't have to just accept what is happening as something you can not do anything about. You also do not need to turn to ineffective methods to help find relief from the symptoms. You can make the choice to implement changes that will help you gain control and allow you to feel at your best for years to come.

The goal of this book is to empower you, encourage you, and support you in the years leading up to, through, and after menopause. You don't have to be taken off guard when the symptoms arise or feel like there is nothing you can do about what is going on. Menopause can be stressful. So many start menopause lost and hopeless. These feelings quickly turn to frustration and disappointment. You don't have to go through this emotional rollercoaster. You embrace menopause from the very beginning without dread.

I have gathered the most valuable information that most women are never taught when it comes to the changes their bodies are going through after they hit 40. Without this knowledge, it is no wonder why many women throw their hands up and just accept their new body, lack of energy, and discomfort as their new normal. You are about to learn that simple lifestyle changes can have a huge impact on symptoms, including weight gain.

This book outlines what to expect when your hormones begin to fluctuate and provides you with an easy-to-use solution to combat the negative effects. You will find four different dieting plans that can help you manage weight and reduce the risk of serious health conditions that most women, over 50, are more concerned about developing. These dieting plans provide you with easy-to-follow guidelines for the best foods to eat, how to get started, and who the diet is best suited for. You will also find meal prepping and recipe ideas that go along with a seven-day meal plan to get started with today. These meal plans are designed to fit into a busy schedule. You won't have to spend every day in the kitchen cooking nutritious meals. Instead, you will see how the meals you prepare can be used throughout the week. This will allow you the freedom to focus on other important activities.

Aside from your diet, you will also understand why it is not too late to start an exercise routine. So many women suffer from age-related bone conditions that occur because of muscle loss and a decrease in bone density. They just accept this as part of the aging process, never realizing that a little extra movement can help combat conditions like osteoporosis. Just because you're older doesn't mean you can't get moving, you are not that old!

Living your best life through menopause is not just about what you eat or how much you exercise. As you will discover, other factors like sleep and stress can contribute to gaining more weight and other health problems. Do not get overwhelmed, however. You may be thinking there are too many changes to make in a short time frame, but this is not the case. Making even a few small changes to your lifestyle can add up to significant changes in the long term.

Menopause lasts for a short time. Usually, within a year you are moving on to the next phase of your life. While menopause will only last this short time, the effects on your health and weight can last for years. You don't need to feel like the extra weight, lack of energy or any of the other age-related conditions that most menopausal women suffer from has to be our fate. You can take control, feel fabulous, and get through menopause in the best shape of your life!

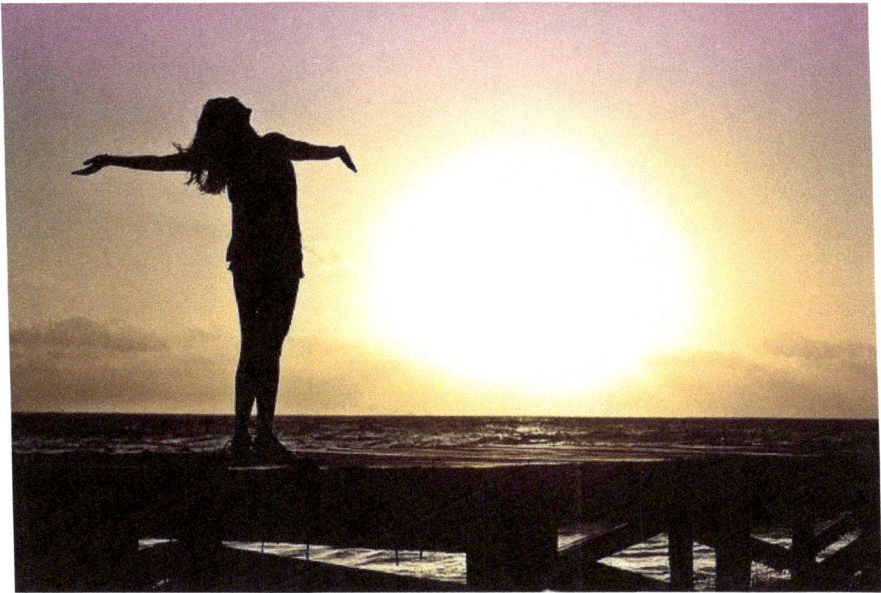

Chapter 1:

Menopause and Weight Struggle

Menopause does not officially start until you have had your last cycle, and, for most women, will last about a year. Menopausal symptoms often begin to occur in the years leading up to menopause, typically around the age of 45. During these transition years, it is not uncommon to experience hot flashes, changes in energy levels, mood swings, and weight gain. Whether you are in the transition phase leading up to menopause or going through menopause it is important to understand what contributes to your symptoms. With this knowledge, you can begin to take action to reverse the effects and feel at your best.

What Causes Weight Gain During Menopause?

There are a few key components that cause older women to gain more weight. Many of these changes, at the time, feel out of your control. You will learn that you can regain control. Just because menopause is a naturally occurring phase, it does not mean you need or should sit back and let the negative effects just happen. Let's first discuss what causes most women to gain weight as they age.

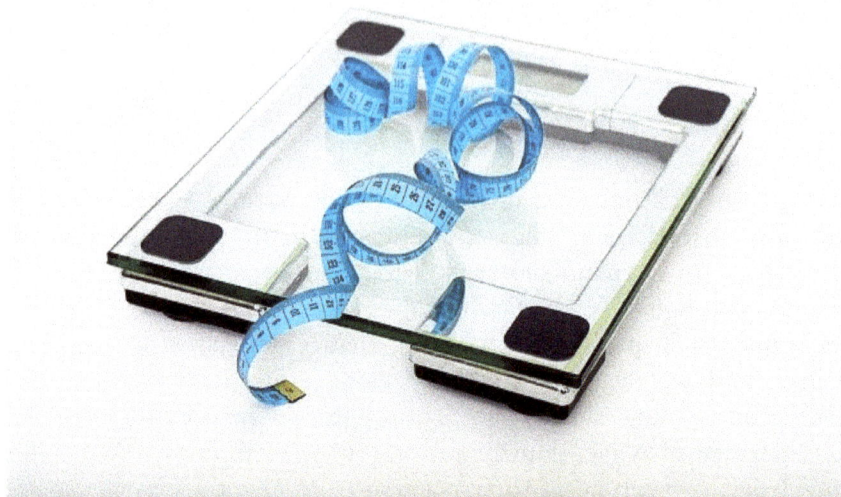

Perimenopause

Perimenopause begins right before menopause starts. For some women this can be in their early 40s, for others it can start in their mid-30s or even early 50s. Perimenopause can last around five to ten years. During perimenopause, you may begin to experience symptoms similar to those of menopause which include:

- hot flashes
- sleep disturbances
- changes to the menstrual cycle
- frequent headaches
- increase irritability
- depression
- anxiety
- weight gain

Gaining excess weight in the perimenopause years will increase the risk of gaining more weight during menopause. Estrogen levels become off-balance during perimenopause which can make it harder to manage your weight. This is also the time when progesterone levels begin to decline. You can begin to combat excess weight gain and other menopausal symptoms during these perimenopausal years.

Change In Hormones

The number one factor that causes women to gain weight during menopause is the change in estrogen levels. Lower estrogen levels during menopause cause visceral fat to build up in the abdomen. Visceral fat puts you at higher risk of insulin resistance, diabetes, and heart disease. This type of fat will begin to form around the organs and can be even more difficult to lose because it is deep below the surface.

Other changes in hormones can cause an increase in appetite because the body feels it needs to be taking in more calories than it actually does. An imbalance in hunger hormones, stress hormones, and appetite-suppressing hormones leads to more weight gain.

Loss of Muscle Mass

The changes in hormones also contribute to a greater loss of muscle mass. This decrease in muscle mass means we feel weaker and will operate at a slower speed. There is also a reduction in bone density. Not only does menopause cause you to lose strength physically, but with weaker bones, we are not able to support as much weight as we used to. These two factors combined put menopausal and post-menopausal women at greater risk of bone-related conditions like osteoporosis.

Metabolism Slows Down

Once again a dip in estrogen is often the blame for a slower metabolic rate during menopause. Your metabolic rate indicates how much energy the body is burning or how much of its stored energy it is converting for working use. However, a decrease in the metabolic rate is a cyclic occurrence. Weight gain can cause estrogen levels to lower, when estrogen levels are low, metabolism slows. When you have a slower metabolism you do not burn as many calories which causes weight gain and therefore causes estrogen levels to drop. This does not mean you have no control over your weight or metabolic rate. During menopause, there are many ways to increase metabolism and shed weight even if your estrogen levels are decreasing.

Age

The average age of women entering menopause is 51. Studies have shown that women who begin menopause before the age of 51 gain less body fat during menopause than women who start after the age of 51 (Spritzler, 2020). A few factors impact this age-related weight gain. As we age, our insulin levels will change. Women entering menopause may have higher fasting insulin levels are more likely to be insulin resistant.

Fasting insulin shows how much insulin is in your blood. Insulin is a hormone that controls glucose or blood sugar levels. This hormone is created by the pancreas and is also used to store extra glucose to convert to energy later. When we have a high fasting insulin level this is often an indicator that the body is not using insulin properly and as a result, we are not using the food we eat properly for energy. High fasting insulin can be a symptom of type 1 or 2 diabetes.

Additionally, losing muscle mass, a slower metabolism, and an increase in fat storage all tend to occur at a more rapid pace as we age. Each of these would contribute to a few extra pounds on their own. During menopause, unfortunately, all these factors seem to bombard us and cause the pounds to just pile on. It does not have to be this way!

Lifestyle

Lifestyle factors play a significant role in how much, if any, the weight you may gain during menopause. Women are at greater risk of becoming obese and developing other serious health conditions during these years. Obesity and cardiovascular disease are avoidable conditions, but you want to be honest about the things you are neglecting that can be putting you at greater risk.

Exercise

Many women decrease their physical activity as they get older. Lack of exercise not only makes it harder to manage weight but can also contribute to the slowing of the metabolism. If you live a more sedentary life, you are going to gain more weight during menopause. Since lean body mass decreases it is more important to make working out a daily routine. Unfortunately, as we get older we are less likely to exercise which only contributes to more weight gain during menopause.

Eating Habits

Diet is another essential element that will cause weight gain. A poor diet will increase the risk of weight gain. Food and drinks that contribute to weight gain even more during menopause include:

- sugar
- alcohol
- salt/sodium
- caffeine

Caffeine and alcohol pose a number of issues during menopause. Both can increase the secretion of cortisol, the stress hormone, that puts you in a fight or flight state. When the body becomes stressed it feels threatened and our natural response to this reaction is to fuel the body in case we need to 'fight'. This response stems back to our early ancestors where they needed to ensure they had enough energy to fight off a predator or flee fast. Since the body's main source of energy comes from carbohydrates you will feel an increase in carb cravings. Carbs often contain a high number of calories.

As you can see, this process is a domino effect that leads to weight gain (increased stress, need for more carbs, higher intake of calories, calories converted to pounds). Additionally, when we consume caffeine or alcohol and this stress response gets triggered our body wants to store its energy as visceral fat. Visceral fat is stored around the organs and is why many women during menopause transition from pear shape to an apple shape in body type and alcohol and caffeine contribute significantly to this fat deposit.

Sleep struggles are often an overlooked factor that can add to weight gain. When we do not get enough sleep our body produces more of the hunger hormone. Getting quality sleep as you enter menopause becomes more of a challenge as our body's heat tolerance changes. You may suffer from hot flashes when you lay down making it feel impossible to sleep comfortably.

Stress Management

Not properly managing stress is another factor that can lead to more weight gain. We addressed what happens when we experience stress while discussing the impact of alcohol and caffeine. Incorporating stress management tools or routines are essential for many reasons, including weight management.

Menopause is a stressful time, and it can also make many women feel isolated and even lost. This is a major life transition that can cause many women to question their life, sort of like a mid-life crisis. It is not uncommon for women to suffer from depression or other mental health issues. These conditions will only contribute to the stress you are already feeling about the changes your body is going through.

What Can You Do About It?

Do not think that just because you cannot control what happens to your dipping estrogen levels you cannot improve your health or feel great through menopause. There are many factors that are within your control that will allow you to breeze through menopause. Now that you have an understanding of what is causing you to gain weight it is time to learn the effective tools that will combat the negative effects you may be experiencing. The remainder of this book will outline how you can lose weight through healthy eating habits. You will discover specific foods that will help minimize menopausal symptoms and what foods to avoid.

You will find some common dieting tips you might have been misguided into believing and why these misconceptions can contribute to poor health and weight gain. You will also find effective ways to address your relationship with foods so you can be sure to fuel your body with nutritious foods. If you do not exercise, you will benefit from the tips on how you can get moving without feeling like you are punishing yourself. You will learn the best types of exercises to perform that will not only slim down your waistline but will build your strength, balance your metabolism, and improve your health. Finally, you will learn additional lifestyle factors that can hinder your weight loss efforts. These additional factors are often neglected but will be easy to address and correct.

You can live your best life during menopause. Let's first get started discussing a few eating plans you want to consider adopting.

Chapter 2:

The Mediterranean Diet for

Menopause

The Mediterranean diet has been ranked as one of the best overall diets for years. It has been researched extensively for its benefits on heart and brain health, but can it help you lose weight, keep it off, and feel great during menopause?

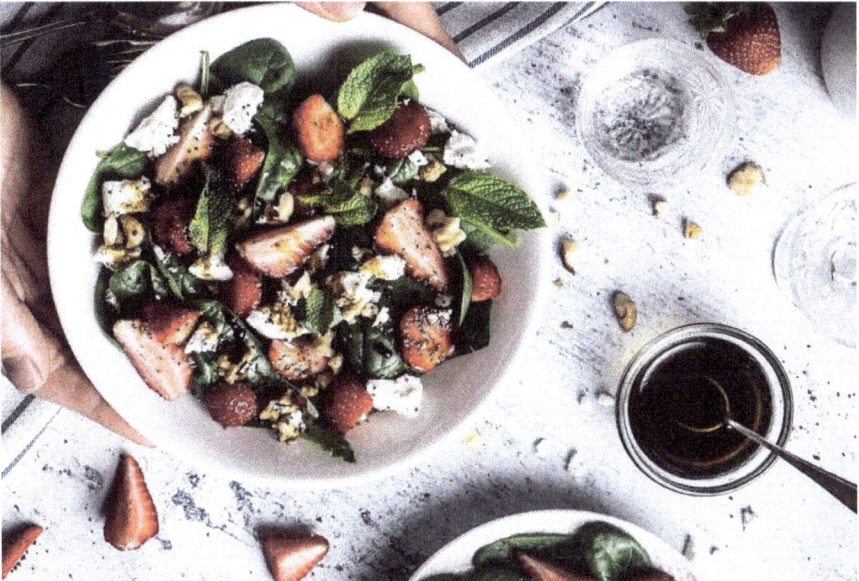

What is the Mediterranean Diet

The Mediterranean diet has been ranked the best diet overall for many years, and for good reason. This diet is flexible and easy to transition to. It was originally designed to model the eating patterns of those living in countries that surround the Mediterranean Sea during the 1950s and 60s. This area was shown to have some of the healthiest populations around the world. Since the people in the area adhered to slightly different diets, you can choose what aspects of the diet to follow. As a general rule, the foods you focus on eating more of include:

- fresh fruits
- fresh vegetables
- fish
- extra virgin olive oil
- whole grains
- nuts
- seeds

There are not many foods that you need to eliminate, but there are some you should avoid, like:

- added sugar
- processed foods
- red meats
- saturated fats

Additionally, you are encouraged to drink a glass of red wine because it contains many antioxidants. However, during menopause, alcohol can cause some symptoms to worsen. You may want to skip the red wine or cut back on how often you have your glass of red.

Aside from what you eat there are a few other things that are encouraged with this diet plan.

1. Get regular exercise. You don't have to work out excessively every day. You should increase your physical activity. Individuals living around the Mediterranean at the time the study conducted on their healthy habits did not rely on cars or other modes of public transportation. Most walked to where they needed to go while others may have had a bike to ride. This physical activity is credited to helping them maintain optimal health.

2. Do not rush through your meals. Meals are meant to be a time to slow down and connect with family and friends. Very rarely will you see individuals walking from one task to another stuffing their face with a doughnut or premade sandwich. Instead, they pause, sit, and enjoy their meals. Don't make eating an afterthought. Mealtimes should be spent connecting with others or simply enjoying your own company.

3. Meal prepping is a part of the process. This connects with the previous content. Meal prepping should also be a time where others help with the cooking of the meal. It is a time to connect with family and friends. It is also a valuable time where everyone in your home can be made to feel they contribute to the household. Even if you are cooking for yourself this is an ideal time to practice some gratitude and bring more awareness to what you are fueling your body with. You will learn later in this book how this can be an important activity that will help you lose weight for good.

How the Mediterranean Diet Helps Weight Loss

The Mediterranean diet does not just focus on changing what you eat. It provides a whole healthy lifestyle solution. When you combine a diet of mostly fruits and vegetables with an increase in physical activity and slowing down, you are taking care of the key aspects of your health—the physical and the mental. While you can certainly lose weight by changing your diet alone you are more likely to maintain a healthy weight with exercise. Those who address their mental stress while trying to lose weight will feel more confident in their abilities to make necessary changes. Additionally, when you get your family and friends involved you have the support to keep you on track with a healthy lifestyle.

This diet is heart health which means it can also help lower the risk of:

- heart disease
- diabetes
- insulin resistance
- cardiovascular disease

The combination of consuming fresh fruits and vegetables along with whole grains has been shown to promote weight loss. These foods are packed with nutrients to keep the body healthy, but also contain high amounts of fiber that help control and combat hunger.

The diet has been studied to show postmenopausal women were able to maintain a higher muscle mass and bone density. This has to do with a combination of changing what they eat and incorporating more physical activity during their day. Exercise is a vital component to staying fit and healthy at any age but is even more important for menopausal women who are prone to lose muscle mass and suffer from osteoporosis.

Aside from health benefits and weight loss, the Mediterranean diet may be able to combat other menopausal symptoms. In one study conducted in Australia, women who follow a Mediterranean diet were less likely to suffer from hot flashes or experience night sweats (Herber-Gast and Mishra, 2013).

Is the Mediterranean Diet Right For You?

Those who want a simple diet plan that requires small changes. Most people do not consider the Mediterranean diet a traditional diet, instead, it is embraced as a lifestyle choice. Because there are no restrictions or set guidelines to follow you can make the Mediterranean eating habit that just becomes a part of who you are. Instead of focusing on foods that are good or bad for you, you are simply encouraged to eat more fruits and vegetables. This is a simple change in what you choose to eat.

Those who want a diet plan that incorporates other aspects of a healthy lifestyle like physical activity. While not a requirement, those who want to start exercising during and after menopause may find the simple approach to increasing physical activity less overwhelming.

This diet is also ideal for those who would rather eat fresh salmon or a big steak. The diet suggests limiting red meat and this should be replaced with fish. If you are not a fan of seafood you might find it harder to reduce the red meat you consume. This is not to say those who do not like fish can not have success with the Mediterranean diet, but those who want to consume more red meat may consider a low-carb or keto diet instead.

Individuals who want to enjoy the foods they eat while still losing weight. There are many flavorful Mediterranean recipes available and it is encouraged that you take the time to savor what you eat.

How To Get Started

Start with one small thing like replacing refined grains with whole grains For example, instead of eating white bread or pasta choose whole wheat or whole-grain bread and pasta.

Fill your plate at least halfway with vegetables. When you start to eat your meals, eat your vegetables first. This will ensure you get the vital nutrient but will also help with your weight loss. Most vegetables are high in fiber, this not only fills you up faster but will keep you feeling full longer. Eating the vegetables first will minimize the risk of overeating at mealtime and in between meals.

Swap out your butter for olive oil. Olive oil is a heart-healthy fat that is consumed freely on the Mediterranean diet. You are best to stick with extra virgin olive oil, which is ideal to consume without being cooked. This oil can add great flavor to many dishes, just drizzle a little overcooked vegetables, dip sourdough bread in it, or use it as a salad dressing.

Speaking of which, instead of store-bought dressing, create your own. Whisk the extra virgin olive oil with herbs and red wine vinegar, white wine vinegar, balsamic vinegar, or apples cider vinegar.

Walk for 20 minutes a day. You do not have to do this all at one. Walk for 10 minutes in the morning then do another 10 minutes later in the day. You can also just find a simple way to increase the steps you take each day. Park further from store entrances, take the stairs, if there is a long way to walk somewhere, take the long way. Incorporating exercise into your daily routine does not have to be the typical "you must hit the gym" to stay in shape. There are plenty of ways you can simply increase the physical activity you already do. We will dive deeper into how to get moving more in Chapter 8.

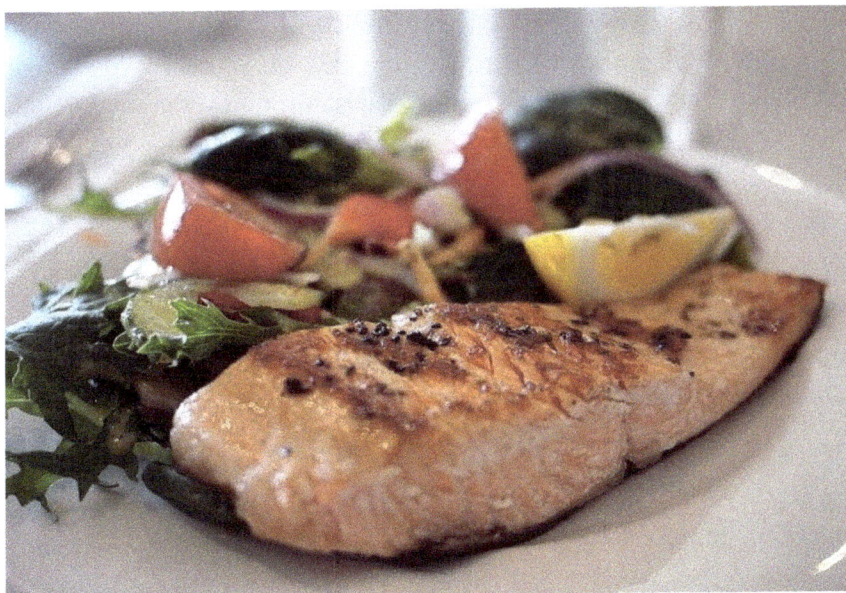

Meal Prep and 7-Day Plan

Recipes and What to Prep

Spinach and Feta Egg Muffins

What you need:

- 12 eggs
- ½ cup soy milk (or regular milk)
- 2 cups spinach (chopped)
- ½ cup feta cheese
- ¼ tsp sea salt
- ¼ tsp black pepper
- olive oil (for greasing muffin tray)

Preheat the oven to 350°F (175°C). Whisk the eggs, milk, salt, and pepper in a mixing bowl. Next, add the spinach and stir. Grease a 12 serving muffin tray with olive oil. Ladle a scoop of the egg mixture into each muffin space. Top with crumbled feta. Bake for 20 minutes or until each muffin has set and is firm yet springy.

This recipe makes six servings (you can have two muffins per serving). Store for up to five days in the fridge. You can use these as breakfast for the week or chop the muffins up and add them to salads.

Blueberry Muffins

What you will need:

- ⅔ cup extra virgin olive oil
- 2 eggs
- 2 cups almond milk
- 2 cups blueberries (if frozen defrost first)
- 2 cups all-purpose flour
- 2 cups whole-wheat flour
- ½ cup sugar
- 6tsp baking powder
- 1 tsp sea salt

Preheat the oven to 400°F (200°C). and grease two 12 servings muffins trays with oil (you can also use a 24 servings tray if you have one). In a medium-size mixing bowl, beat the eggs and milk, then add the olive oil and mix thoroughly. Set aside. Take a large mixing bowl and add the flours, sugar, baking powder, and salt. Use a fork to mix everything. Add the wet ingredients into the large bowl with the dry ingredients. Stir until everything is thoroughly incorporated then fold in the blueberries. Ladle the mixture into the muffin trays. Bake for 18 minutes or until the centers are cooked through, test with a toothpick.

This recipe makes 24 muffins. The meal plan uses them as breakfast options but you can also have them as an after-dinner treat. You can keep the muffins in the fridge for up to seven days.

Greek Salad

What you will need:

- 4 tbsp extra virgin olive oil
- ½ cup cherry tomatoes (cut in half)
- 1 cucumber (chopped)
- 2 cups spinach
- 12 Kalamata olives
- ¼ cup feta cheese crumbles
- 2 tbsp red wine vinegar or freshly squeezed lemon juice
- 1 tbsp oregano (dried)

Toss the tomatoes, cucumber, spinach, and olives in a large salad bowl. Whisk the olive oil and red wine vinegar in a small mixing bowl. Pour over the salad and toss, then sprinkle on the feta cheese crumbles. This recipe will be used as a side dish for one dinner and one lunch option. You can also choose to use it as four lunch options during the week. The salad will stay fresh in the fridge for up to five days.

Mushroom, Spinach, and Penne Soup

What you will need:

- 4 tbsp olive oil
- 3 cups penne pasta
- 4 cups vegetable broth
- 1 cup heavy cream
- 1 cup porcini mushrooms (diced)
- 1 cup shiitake mushrooms (diced)
- 2 garlic cloves (minced)
- 4 cups spinach (chopped)
- 2 tbsp thyme (chopped)
- 2 tbsp oregano (chopped)
- 2 tbsp parsley (chopped)
- ½ cup parmesan cheese (grated)

- ¼ tsp sea salt
- ¼ tsp black pepper

Place a large dutch oven pot on the stove over medium heat. Add the olive oil, once the oil is warm add the garlic. Cook for two minutes, then add the thyme, oregano, and parsley. Stir and cook for two more minutes. Pour in the chicken broth and allow it to come to a boil. Add the mushrooms, pasta, and parmesan cheese, lower the heat to medium-low, and simmer for 10 minutes. Next, add spinach, heavy cream, salt, and pepper. Cook for five more minutes then serve.

This recipe makes six servings. The meal plan uses the soup as a lunch option but you can also serve it as a dinner option and use leftovers as lunch for the week. Store in the refrigerator for up to seven days.

Tofu Coconut Curry

What you will need:

- 2 tbsp coconut oil
- 1 15-ounce can of coconut milk
- 12-ounce block of firm tofu (pat dry, cubed)
- 2 carrots (peeled, sliced)
- 1 red bell pepper (cubed)
- 1 cup snap peas
- 1 onion (diced)
- 2 garlic cloves (minced)
- ½-inch piece of ginger (minced)
- 1 tbsp red Thai curry paste (more if desired)
- 1 tsp fish sauce
- ¼ tsp salt
- 1 cup basmati rice

Bring two cups of water to a boil in a medium-size pot, then add the rice. Stir, cover, and simmer for 15 minutes. As the rice cooks, heat one tablespoon of coconut oil in a large skillet. Once the oil has melted, add the tofu to the oil and cook for two minutes on each side or until crispy. You will have to fry the tofu in batches. Once the tofu has been cooked add another tablespoon of coconut oil to the same pan. Add the onions, carrots, and red bell pepper, cook for five minutes stirring occasionally.

Next, add the ginger and garlic to the pan. Cook for one minute then stir in the curry paste, be sure that all the vegetables are nicely coated. Pour over the coconut milk and stir with a wooden spoon. Make sure you scrap the button of the pan to loosen up all the flavorful little bits. Add the fish sauce, stir, and taste to see if you would like to add more curry paste. Finally, add the crispy tofu, snow peas, and sea salt. Lower the heat and simmer for 10 minutes, stirring occasionally. Serve the curry with basmati rice.

This recipe makes four servings. For the meal plan, you will see this as one dinner and one lunch option but you can easily use this just for four lunch options to minimize the cooking during the week.

Sheet Pan Chicken with Peppers and Onions

What you will need:
- ¼ cup olive oil plus extra for drizzling over the chicken
- 4 chicken thighs (skin on)
- 2 red bell peppers
- 2 yellow bell peppers
- 2 vidalia onions (sliced)
- 2 garlic cloves (chopped)
- 1 15-ounce can fire-roasted diced tomatoes
- 1 tsp paprika
- ½ tsp oregano
- ½ tsp basil
- ½ tsp sea salt (divided)
- ½ tsp black pepper (divided)

Preheat the oven to 400°F (200°C). Arrange the peppers, onions, and garlic in a single layer on a large sheet pan. Pour the ¼ olive oil over the vegetables and the can of fire-roasted tomatoes. Toss lightly then sprinkle with ¼ teaspoon of sea salt and pepper. Set the vegetables aside. Drizzle a little of the olive oil over the chicken and sprinkle with ¼ teaspoon of sea salt and pepper. Set the chicken on top of the peppers and onions. Sprinkle the oregano, basil, and paprika over the top of everything. Bake for one hour and fifteen minutes.

This recipe makes four servings and will be used for one dinner and one lunch option in the meal plan. Store in the fridge for up to five days. You can also store it in the freezer for up to three months.

Meal Plan

Monday

Breakfast: Spinach and Feta egg muffin with whole wheat toast and a banana.

Lunch: Mushroom, spinach, and penne soup.

Dinner: Tofu coconut curry.

Tuesday

Breakfast: Blueberry muffins and sliced melon.

Lunch: Mushroom, spinach, and penne soup.

Dinner: Herbs crusted salmon with roasted small potatoes and Greek salad.

Wednesday

Breakfast: Oatmeal with cinnamon and apples.

Lunch: Leftover tofu coconut curry.

Dinner: Sheet Pan Chicken with Peppers and Onions.

Thursday

Breakfast: Green smoothie: Blend 1 ½ cups almond milk, a cup of spinach, a fourth an avocado, ½ cup of mixed berries (frozen or fresh), a clementine (peel removed), 5 walnuts, 1 tablespoon each of chia seed and flaxseed.

Lunch: Leftover Greek salad.

Dinner: Spaghetti squash with bolognese sauce.

Friday

Breakfast: Blueberry muffins and a cup of Greek yogurt.

Lunch: Leftover sheet pan chicken with peppers and onions and quinoa.

Dinner: Baked cod with spinach, olive, and sun-dried tomato salad.

Saturday

Breakfast: Fruit smoothie: Blend a cup of pineapple chunks, a Pink lady apple (core and seeds removed), ½ a banana (frozen), ½ cup plain Greek yogurt, a tablespoon of coconut oil, a tablespoon each of chia seed and flaxseed, and a cup of coconut water.

Lunch: Mushroom, spinach, and penne soup.

Dinner: Vegetable kebabs and whole wheat pita served with a mixed green salad.

Sunday

Breakfast: Scrambled eggs and a blueberry muffin.

Lunch: Mushroom, spinach, and penne soup.

Dinner: Grilled salmon: Rub 2 salmon filets with a tablespoon of each; olive oil, red wine vinegar, and capers. Grill the salmon for 8 minutes (skin side down). Serve with boiled potatoes and corn on the cob.

Chapter 3:

Low-Carb Diet for Menopause

During menopause, the body changes in how it uses food for energy. Many women find that the carbs they eat are adding more weight without providing them more energy. A low-carb diet may help the body use the foods you eat in a more effective manner. Some low-carb diets trigger the body to burn through more stored fat, while others help you reduce your caloric intake daily. There are no one-size-fits-all when it comes to low-carb dieting, which is why many women favor this eating plan. You can customize a low-carb diet to suit your preferences, weight loss, and health goals.

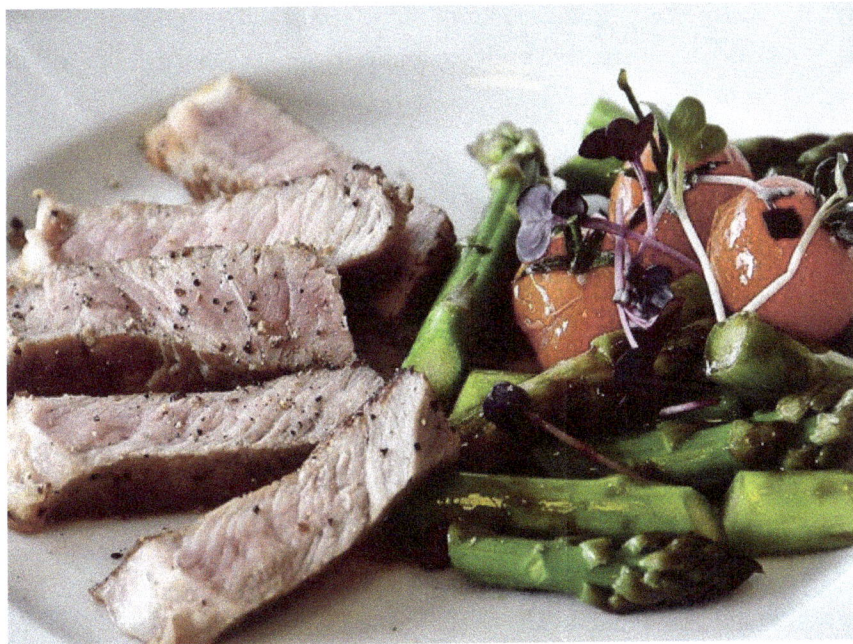

What is a Low-Carb Diet

It is recommended that we consume between 225 to 325 g of carbs a day, but most consume significantly more than this. A low-carb diet cuts this carb intake in half and sometimes more.

There are many variations of a low-carb diet such as:

- Atkin: A four-phase low-carb diet that first minimizes carbs to just 20 grams a day for two weeks. Then you begin to add low-carb foods (vegetables, nuts, fruits) back to your diet. The third is where you fine-tune your diet plan. This phase is when weight loss will slow down as you get closer to your target weight. The final phase is focused on maintaining your new weight.

- Keto: Very low-carb and high-fat diet. Designed to trigger ketosis where the body naturally begins to burn more of its stored fat as fuel.

- Paleo- This diet is naturally low-carb as it focuses on eating fresh fruits, vegetables, lean meats, nuts, and seeds. It eliminates many processed foods that tend to be much higher in carbs and calories.

Many other diets have been modified to fit into a low-carb profile, such as a low-carb Mediterranean diet.

Overall, any diet can be considered low-carb as long as you are eating fewer carbs than you typically would. Many of these types of diets will have specific recommendations for carb intake. The Keto Diet for example restricts carb intake to no more than 50 grams a day and ideally encourages individuals to stick to under 30 grams a day.

A basic low-carb diet sets a goal for under 100 grams but no lower than 50 grams. An easy way to approach a low carb diet is:

- For rapid weight loss restrict carbs to 50 grams or fewer carbs a day.
- For a steady approach to weight loss, keep carbohydrates between 50 to 100 grams a day.
- To maintain your ideal weight limit carbs to between 100 and 150 grams a day.

A low-carb diet can be flexible and those going through menopause may benefit greatly from consuming fewer calories. Unless you are following a strict low-carb diet like the Keto plan or Atkins there are not many restrictions on a low-carb diet.

On a standard low-carb diet, you focus on eating more:

- animal proteins
- fats
- non-starchy vegetables
- full-fat dairy
- nuts and seeds

Plant proteins should also be included but only moderately. These include legumes, beans, and soy.

While not completely eliminated on a standard low-carb diet there are foods you want to consume minimally such as fruits, starchy vegetables, and whole grains. Foods you are strongly encouraged to eliminate from your diet include:

- sugars (including natural sugar and added sugars)
- processed foods
- refined grains
- low fat or diet foods

When going with a low-carb diet you want to ensure you are getting enough fiber. This is vital for keeping the digestive tract healthy but will also aid in your weight loss efforts. Most fruits are high in fiber, but since it is recommended that you limit your consumption of fruit because of their high carb count, you need to find your fiber from another source. Broccoli, lentils, and some beans can be a great choice for fiber, but remember this is something you need to consume daily.

How A Low-Carb Diet Helps Weight Loss

Several studies show the impact of a low-carb diet and weight gain during menopause. One study that involved more than 88,000 participants showed that women on a low-carb diet gain less weight during menopause than women on other types of diet plans (Link and Northrop, 2020). Keep in mind that this low-carb diet was specifically a Keto diet where carb restriction is limited significantly to just 50 grams or less a day. This does not mean that you will still not have success with a low-carb diet, it is just to make you aware of the difference in carb restrictions.

Many carbohydrate-rich foods contain a higher amount of calories. If we want to lose weight we know we need to have a caloric deficit so that our body is burning more calories throughout the day than we are giving it. Cutting out carbohydrates for most will naturally lead to consuming fewer calories which helps the weight come off. By restricting carb intake we allow the body to burn up its stored fat. This is the driving factor behind the keto diet.

The body's main source of fuel is carbohydrates and carbs come in many forms: whole grains, processed flour, and sugar. The body converts carbohydrates into glucose and this glucose is distributed to the cells in the body for fuel. If we take in more carbohydrates than our body needs the excess gets converted to fat and is stored for later use. Unfortunately, because most individuals consume way more carbs throughout the day then the body can use most of what we eat gets stored away. The body does not access this stored fat for fuel because we supply it with a constant stream of fuel from carbohydrates. Cutting out the instant fuel source (carbohydrates) we trigger the body to utilize the stored fat as fuel instead through ketosis. This is a natural process the body is designed to perform but, as mentioned, is not something our body is used to doing because our diets typically keep the carbs flowing.

Is a Low Carb Diet Right for You?

Cutting back on carbs is a great idea especially if you consume a high amount of carbs already. You do not need to stick to an extremely low, low-carb diet like the Keto Diet. For many women, sticking to a low-carb diet that restricts carbs to under 100 grams a day can help lose unwanted weight but, there is a greater risk of gaining the weight back. A low-carb diet is ideal for those who can keep their carb intake to a manageable level, between 150 to 250 grams a day.

Menopause puts women at a higher risk of heart disease. Since a low-carb diet often encourages increased fat intake this can put you at even more risk. It is important that the fats you include in your diet are healthy fats such as those from vegetable oils like extra virgin olive oil and avocado.

It is important to discuss your dietary changes with your healthcare provider. Then can go over your risk of developing certain conditions and help you determine if a low-carb diet is beneficial for you. Again, a low-carb diet is simply cutting back on your carb intake and increasing your consumption of whole foods.

Getting Started Tips

Try not to get caught up on which type of low-carb diet you want to try. Whether you label it Keto or Paleo your focus should be the same; eat more whole foods. You can transition to a low-carb diet by simply eating fewer carbs than you currently do. Cutting back on carb intake so that you are getting the daily recommendation of around 225g can have a serious positive impact on your weight and health. If you are one of the few who already meet this daily requirement then consider cutting back just a little more.

Track your carb intake so you have a realistic idea of how many carbs you are consuming daily. Cutting back on carbs will be much easier when you have a clear outline of where you can cut them from. Many people do not realize just how many breads, pastas, and grains they consume throughout the day. When you track what you are eating for at least a week you will find that you swap out some of those carbs for more vegetables or lean meats.

While a low-carb diet can jumpstart your weight loss efforts, following a low-carb diet that restricts carb intake to under 100g a day can have negative effects on one's health. Studies indicate that a diet that restricts carbs significantly like this for a prolonged time can increase the risk of health conditions like cardiovascular disease and heart disease. For weight loss, you can restrict carbs significantly, but once you reach your ideal weight you want to reintroduce more carbs into your diet. This can be tricky as you need to add in more carbs slowly to ensure you are keeping the weight off. It is always best to stick with starchy vegetables and whole grains when you increase your carb intake. These will provide you with what you need along with additional nutrients that will keep your health in great standing.

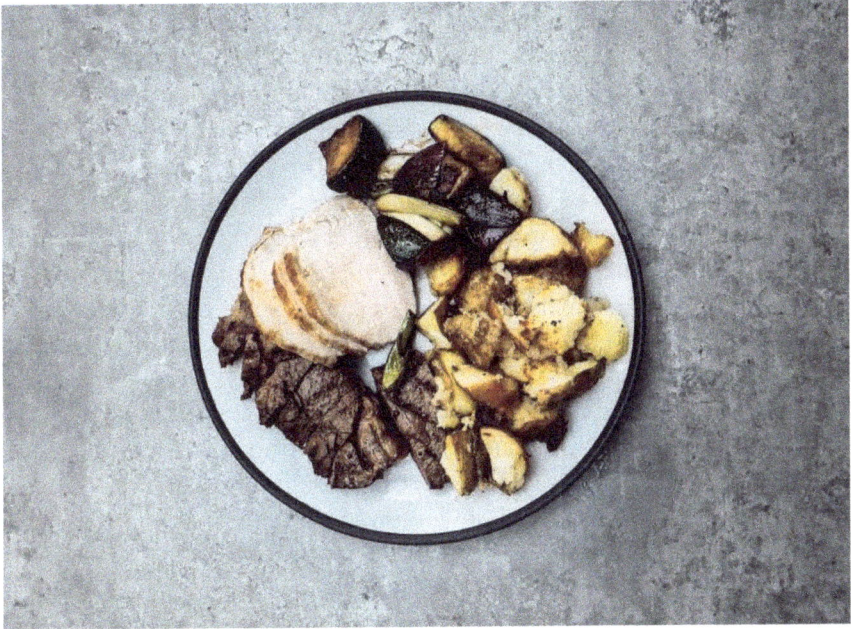

Meal Prep and 7-Day Plan

Recipes and What to Prep

Cloud Bread

What you will need:

- 3 eggs (separate egg whites from the yolks)
- ½ cup cream cheese
- ½ tbsp ground flaxseed
- 1 tsp baking powder
- ¼ tsp cream of tartar
- ¼ tsp sea salt

Preheat your oven to 350°F (175°C). Line a baking sheet with parchment paper and set the sheet aside. In a metal bowl whip the egg whites, salt, and cream of tartar. The egg whites should be stiff and when you flip the bowl over the eggs whites will remain in the bowl. Take another small mixing bowl and whisk the egg yolk, cream cheese, ground flaxseed, and baking powder, Carefully fold the egg yolk into the egg whites. Scoop a spoonful of the egg mixture onto the baking sheet with parchment paper. Gently spread the mixture into a circle that is about ½-inch thick. You should have four circles. Bake for 25 minutes or until the eggs turn a light golden color.

This recipe makes two servings. You can store the bread in the refrigerator for up to three days. They can also be stored in the freezer for up to three months. To store, place parchment paper in between the bread pieces. To reheat, form the freeze in the oven for five minutes at 300°F.

Bacon and Egg Muffins

What you will need:

- 12 eggs
- 5 oz bacon (cooked, chopped)
- 2 scallions (chopped fine)
- 2 tbsp green pesto
- 1 ½ cups cheddar cheese (shredded)
- ¼ tsp sea salt
- ¼ tsp black pepper

Preheat the oven to 300°F (150°C) and a 12 servings muffin tray with baking cups or liners. You can also grease a silicone muffin mold if you have one. Place the chopped scallions and bacon in the bottom of each muffin section. In a medium-size mixing bowl whisk the eggs with the pesto, cheddar cheese, salt, and pepper. Once thoroughly combined, transfer the egg mixture into the muffin tray, pouring it over the scallion and bacon. Set the muffin tray in the oven and bake for 15 minutes or until the eggs start to turn a golden brown.

This recipe makes six servings (two muffins per serving). They will stay fresh in the fridge for up to four days or you can freeze them for up to three months.

Bunless Burger Patties

What you will need:

- 1 ½ lbs ground chicken or beef
- 1 egg
- 1 scallion (diced fine)
- 1 garlic clove (minced)
- ½ tsp sea salt
- ½ tsp black pepper

In a large mixing bowl use your hands to combine the ground chicken, egg, dice scallion, garlic, salt, and pepper. Divide the mixture into four equal portions and shape it into burger patties. Place a large skillet on the stove over high heat. Once the pan is hot, lower the heat to medium and place the burger patties in it, cook on each side for five minutes or until the patties turn a dark golden brown.

This recipe makes four servings. You can use this as a dinner option, the sample meal plan uses this recipe as lunch during the week. These patties are served on two large lettuce leaves with sliced tomatoes, avocado, and onions. You can serve them with a side salad or sweet potato fries. Store the patties in the refrigerator for up to five days. They can also be kept in the freezer for up to three months. Be sure to wrap the patties individually when storing them in the freezer.

Zucchini Pizza

What you will need for the crust:

- 2 eggs
- 1 ½ lbs zucchini (shredded, and squeezed to release excess water)

- 1 cup shredded cheese
- 1 tsp baking powder
- 1 tsp dried oregano
- 1 tsp black pepper

For toppings you will need:

- ½ cup tomato sauce
- 2 cups shredded mozzarella
- 3 oz pepperoni
- ¾ cup sliced green bell pepper
- 1 tbsp dried basil

Preheat the oven to 425°F (220°C) and line a baking sheet with parchment paper, then set it to the side. Mix all the crust ingredients in a large mixing bowl until you have a smooth batter. Spread the batter onto the lined baking sheet. Smooth the batter out using a rubber spatula to form the crust of the pizza. Place in the oven for 15 minutes or until the crust turns a light golden brown. Take the crust out of the oven. Spread the tomato sauce then sprinkle over the cheese. Add the pepperoni and bell pepper, then spank the dried basil over the top of everything. Place back in the oven and back for another 15 minutes or until the cheese is completely melted. Allow the pizza to cool slightly before slicing.

These recipes should serve four. You will see this used as a dinner option and two lunch options in the sample menu. If you are cooking dinner for more than yourself you want to double the recipe and make two so you have enough for lunch. Store leftovers for up to five days in your refrigerator.

Shrimp and Cabbage

What you will need:

- 4 tbsp coconut oil (divided)
- 1 ½ lbs jump shrimp (peeled, deveined, leave the tail on)
- 2 lbs cabbage (sliced)

- 4 garlic cloves (chopped)
- 2 limes (juice only)
- 2 tbsp fresh ginger (chopped fine)
- 4 tbsp tamari soy sauce
- 1 cup fresh cilantro (chopped)
- 4 tbsp sesame seeds
- ½ tsp sea salt
- ¼ tsp black pepper

Place two tablespoons of coconut oil in a large frying pan or wok. Add the shredded cabbage, garlic, and ginger. Cook for one minute, then add a splash of water and cook until the cabbage becomes tender, stirring occasionally. Add the soy sauce, lime juice, sesame seed, and cilantro. Turn the heat to low, stir occasionally, and cook until ready to serve. In a separate frying pan add the other two tablespoons of coconut nut oil. Turn the heat to medium, when the oil has melted add the shrimp. Sprinkle it with salt and pepper. Cook for three minutes, flip, and cook for another three minutes or until the shrimp is no longer translucent. Serve the shrimp over top of the cabbage mixture and garnish it with fresh cilantro.

This recipe makes four servings. It is used as a dinner option and one lunch option. Store any leftovers for five days in your fridge.

Chicken Stir Fry with Broccoli and Snow Peas

What you will need:

- 2 tbsp coconut oil
- 2 tbsp tamari soy sauce
- 2 lbs boneless chicken thighs (sliced thin)
- 3 cups broccoli (cut to bite-size pieces)
- 1 cup snow peas
- 2 garlic cloves (minced)
- 1 tsp garlic powder
- 1 tsp black pepper

Add the oil to a large frying pan or wok. Turn the heat to medium-high. Once the oil has melted, add the sliced chicken, garlic powder, black pepper. Cook for 10 minutes or until the chicken has turned a light brown. Next, add the broccoli and soy sauce. Stir, and cook for five minutes. Next, add the garlic and snow peas. Cook for another five minutes then serve.

This recipe makes four servings and is used as one dinner option and one lunch option in the meal plan. Store your leftovers in the fridge for not more than five days.

Low-Carb Snack Ideas:

You can incorporate two snacks a day with a low-carb diet, usually one snack between breakfast and lunch and another between lunch and dinner. Some ideas to try include:

- vegetable sticks and hummus
- mini bell pepper with cream cheese or hummus
- apple slice and nut butter
- a handful of mixed nuts
- turkey and cheese rolls
- vegetables stick rolls (rolled in lettuce leaves and topped with hummus)
- avocado and tomato slices on cloud bread
- greek yogurt
- cottage cheese
- string cheese

Meal Plan

Monday

Breakfast: Bacon, lettuce, tomato, and mayo on cloud bread.

Lunch: Bunless burger served on a large lettuce leaf with tomatoes, avocado, onion slices.

Dinner: Shrimp and cabbage.

Tuesday

Breakfast: Bacon and egg muffins.

Lunch: Leftover shrimp and cabbage with spinach and cherry tomatoes.

Dinner: Zucchini pizza.

Wednesday

Breakfast: Bacon and egg muffins.

Lunch: Bunless burger served on a large lettuce leaf with tomato, avocado, and onion slices.

Dinner: Low-carb chicken parmesan.

Thursday

Breakfast: Two fried eggs with a side of spinach, tomato, avocado.

Lunch: Zucchini pizza.

Dinner: Taco salad: made with ground beef, lettuce, black beans, cheddar cheese and topped with salsa and guacamole.

Friday

Breakfast: Bacon and egg muffins.

Lunch: Bunless burger served on a large lettuce leaf with tomato, avocado, and onion slices.

Dinner: Vegetable soup.

Saturday

Breakfast: Mushroom and onion omelet.

Lunch: Zucchini pizza.

Dinner: Chicken stir fry with broccoli and snow peas.

Sunday

Breakfast: Scrambled eggs with a side of watermelon.

Lunch: Leftover chicken stir fry with broccoli and snow peas.

Dinner: Zucchini lasagna.

Chapter 4:

Vegan and Vegetarian Diet for

Menopause

Eating a diet full of fruits and vegetables will improve your overall health and help you lose weight without depriving the body of what it needs. There are many variations to a vegetarian diet. Some people stick with this type of eating plan for most days of the week and allow themselves lean cuts of meat once or twice a week. Others, only eat specific types of animal products like eggs or fish. You can tailor a vegetarian diet to your preferences and still benefit from the extra fruits and vegetables you consume. Learn how a vegan or vegetarian diet can help you lose weight during menopause and beyond.

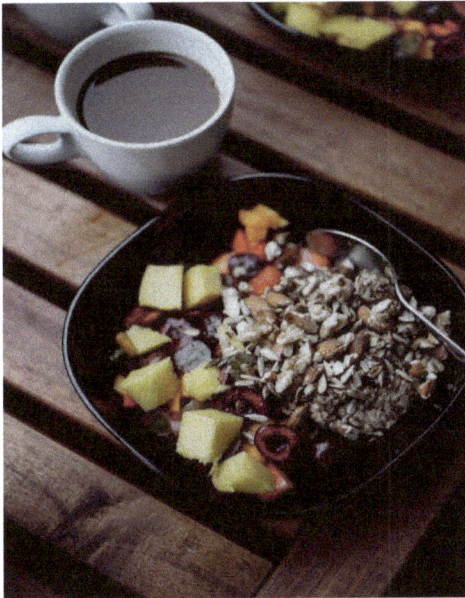

What is a Vegan and Vegetarian Diet

There is more than one way to stick with a vegetarian diet. Different types of vegetarian diets include:

- Traditional vegetarian: This type of vegetarian diet excludes all meat, poultry, and fish. Those who are traditional vegetarians may still incorporate animal-derived products like honey and some dairy like milk or cheese.

- Ovo-Vegetarian: An Ovo-vegetarian excludes all meat, poultry, seafood, and eggs. Those on this type of vegetarian diet will eat eggs.

- Lacto-Vegetarian: A Lacto-vegetarian will again exclude all meat, poultry, seafood. They will not eat eggs but will include dairy products.

- Lacto Ovo Vegetarian: Lacto Ovo vegetarians are a combination of both, Lacto and Ovo-vegetarians. They allow for dairy and eggs, but still exclude all meat, poultry, and seafood.

- Vegan: A vegan strictly cuts out all animal products and animal by-products. they will not consume any meat, seafood, poultry, dairy, eggs, or honey.

As you can see a vegetarian diet can be flexible to include some additional proteins and calcium-rich foods in your diet which is essential for maintaining proper health. Whether you choose to go all vegan or stick with another variation of vegetarian the main foods you will be eating are plant-based—fruits, vegetables, whole grains.

What makes vegetarianism or veganism more complex is knowing how to buy outside of these three main groups. Buying packaged foods, including sauces and condiments, requires a clear understanding of how to read food labels. Many ingredients added to various products in the supermarket include animal by-products. Gelatin is a prime example of this, but eggs and milk are also well-known ingredients in many packaged products.

Vegetarians and vegans will not eat any animal products like red meat and poultry. However, you do get to decide if you want to include dairy products in your diet. Another item to be aware of is that most vegans exclude honey or other bee products from their diet, while vegetarians find this to be ok to consume. There is no right or wrong approach to becoming vegetarian or vegan, this is why many people enjoy this eating plan; it is also for flexibility.

One thing to mention, however, is to be aware when buying 'vegan' products. Since this eating style has become more popular many companies have manufactured products to appeal to these individuals, Vegan cheese, vegan turkey, and vegan butter, allowing you to enjoy the same flavor as these non-vegan products, but this does not mean they are the best option for you. Most vegan products will have additives and be highly processed to provide enjoyable flavors. They may also be lacking nutrients that you could get from other natural products. Be mindful of how much and how often you consume these vegan products.

How a Vegan or Vegetarian Diet Helps Weight Loss

A diet that focuses on eating more fruits and vegetables will result in weight loss. During menopause, studies have shown women who stuck to a vegetarian diet with no calories restriction lost over seven pounds more than women who adhered to a diet that include more animal products (Barnard et al., 2015). Other studies have shown that post-menopausal women who adopted a vegan diet lost more weight overall than those following an omnivore diet (Beezhold et al., 2018).

Vegetarian and vegan diets incorporate more soy than many other diet plans. Studies show that a plant-based diet that includes soy products can help women during menopause avoid hot flashes. The Women's Study for the Alleviation of Vasomotor Symptoms study showed that women on a plant-based diet that incorporate soy saw a reduction of hot flash symptoms by 79%, and nearly 60% of the participants confirmed that after the 12-week study they experienced no hot flashes (Barnard et al., 2021).

Is a Vegan or Vegetarian Diet Right For You?

Even if you are not keen on cutting out all animal products there are ways you can be vegan or vegetarian part of the time and still receive some of the benefits from this diet. Many women choose to stick to a vegan or vegetarian diet five days a week but allow themselves more freedom on the weekends. This is not the type of diet you need to fully commit to. Some aspects of the diet you do, however, want to commit to daily. Cutting out processed foods and sticking to more plant-based, whole foods will provide you with the most benefits during menopause.

Women who embraced a vegan or vegetarian diet for at least most days of the week have more success with sticking to this way of eating for the long term, not just to lose weight. When you can maintain your eating habits for life, you will continue to reap the benefits which means the weight you lose will stay off.

If you desire a flexible and easy-to-maintain diet, a vegan or vegetarian eating plan may be the best fit for you. You can slowly transition to vegetarianism over time until you are eating very little to no animal products. With an approach like this, where you do not have to make many changes all at once, you are more likely to have success sticking to this eating plan for the long term.

Getting Started Tips

Know how to get adequate protein into your diet. Plant-based proteins include lentils, beans, nuts, and seeds. Additionally, you can incorporate other protein sources like tofu, tempeh, and soy-based products.

The following are additional nutrients you want to ensure you are getting enough of:

- Vitamin B12. The body requires vitamin B12 to produce red blood cells and reduce the risk of developing anemia. Unfortunately, vitamin B12 is only obtained naturally through the consumption of animal products. Vegetarians and vegans need to choose vitamin-enriched cereals that contain vitamin B12 and soy products that have added B12 to them.

- Vitamin D. Getting enough vitamin D in your diet is essential for bone health. As we get older it can become more difficult for the body to absorb enough vitamin D. Sunlight exposure is the best source of vitamin D, but you may live in an area that does not get adequate sunlight to ensure you absorb enough vitamin D. Other sources of vitamin D include soy milk, rice milk, and fortified cereals. It may be necessary to take a vitamin D supplement which you want to ensure is derived from plants.

- Zinc. There are many enzymes in the body that rely on zinc and it is also essential for creating protein and performing cell division in the body. Zinc can be obtained through cheese but can also be found in legumes, nuts, whole grains, and soy.

- Calcium. We know we need plenty of calcium to maintain healthy bones and teeth. Aside from dairy, collard greens, broccoli, and kale will provide you with calcium. You can also choose calcium-rich, fortified foods like soy milk, tofu, and cereals.

- Iron. Iron is essential for their health and production of red blood cells. Many plant-based sources contain iron. Beans, lentils, dark leafy greens, whole grains, and dried foods contain iron. The body needs vitamin C to absorb iron so be sure to include plenty of vitamin C-rich foods like citrus fruits, cabbage, and berries, into your diet as well.

- Omega-3 fatty acids. These essential acids maintain heart and brain health. and the best way to obtain omega-3 fatty acids is through wild-caught fish and eggs. Other foods that can provide you with a little omega-3 fatty acid include canola oil, soy oil, flaxseeds, walnuts, and soybeans. Keep in mind, however, that these plant-based sources may not convert as easily or properly in the body as the omega-3 obtained through fish and eggs. You may want to consider a plant-based omega-3 supplement or choose fortified products that contain omega-3s.

- Iodine. Iodine is often neglected when it comes to the essential nutrients your body needs but is especially important for older women. Iodine plays a vital role in thyroid hormones which are responsible for regulating metabolism. Many vegans and vegetarians do not get enough iodine in their diet. Even worse, those who consume excess soy, sweet potatoes, and cruciferous vegetables like broccoli are at an even greater risk of iodine deficiency which can lead to goiter or irregular growth of the thyroid gland. Luckily, you can ensure you get enough iodine in your diet by consuming a ¼ a teaspoon of iodized salt daily.

Do not get trapped into vegan labels. As mentioned, vegan products do not always mean better for you. When shopping for the best vegan foods read the labels and be aware of added sugars, salt, and highly processed foods. As a general rule, if a product contains too many words you cannot pronounce in the ingredients list it is best to avoid it. Another rule to stick with when shopping for plant-based products is to choose products that have a short list of ingredients. If there are more than five ingredients on the list there is a greater chance that it will contain unhealthy items that won't help you lose weight or keep it off, and can increase other menopause symptoms.

Experiment with different recipes, herbs, spices, and sauces. There are plenty of plant-based recipes you can find online and even more cookbooks available that are purely plant-based. Don't think your meals have to be bland and boring. Trying new recipes will keep your diet fun and exciting!

Stick with a meatless plan that you can commit to. As mentioned you do not have to go all in, you can slowly begin to cut down on your animal product intake one day at a time. Meatless Mondays are a popular approach to transitioning to vegetarianism. Remember, a successful diet that helps you lose weight and keep it off is one you can incorporate as a lifestyle choice. You may not want to go fully vegetarian or vegan but can go meatless three or more days a week. Do what world for you.

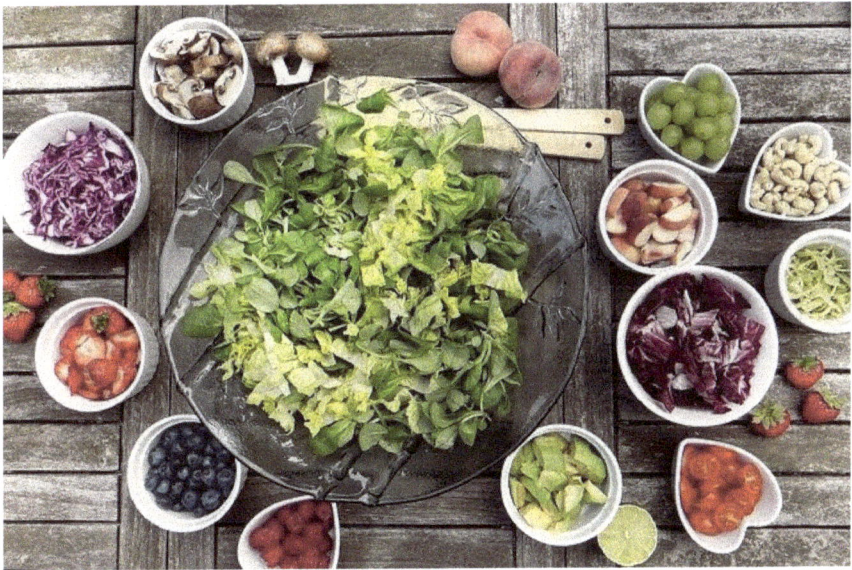

Meal Prep and 7-Day Plan

Recipes and What to Prep

Tofu Scramble

What you will need:

- 1 tbsp coconut oil
- 16 oz block of firm tofu, cut into 1-inch cubes
- 1 onion finely chopped
- 2 tomatoes, diced
- 1 tsp dried basil
- 1 tsp turmeric
- 2 tbsp soya sauce

Place the coconut oil, basil, and turmeric in a pan and cook over medium heat for five minutes. Stir frequently to avoid burning, then add the onions and saute until they become translucent. Add the tofu cubes and use a wooden spatula to break up the pieces so you have a scrambled egg texture. Cook the tofu for five minutes, then add the tomatoes and soya sauce. Stir and cook for another five minutes.

Divide the mixture into four equal servings and store in an airtight container for breakfast during the week.

Sweet Potato Waffles

What you will need:

- Cooking spray to spray the waffle maker
- ¾ cup oats
- 1 large sweet potato (this should equal 1 ½ cups of cooked slightly mashed potatoes)

- ½ cup almond flour
- ¾ cup almond milk
- 6 tbsp applesauce
- 1 tbsp baking powder
- 1 tsp cinnamon
- ¼ tsp sea salt

As your waffle maker heats up, place the cooked sweet potato and oats into a blender. Pulse a few times to break everything up, then add the remaining ingredients. Blend until smooth, be sure to pause two or three times and scrape the sides to get all the chunks out. After the waffle maker is hot, spray it with cooking spray, then ladle the sweet potato batter onto the maker. Close and cook for 10 minutes. Remove and enjoy with pure maple syrup, fresh berries, and coconut whipped cream.

This recipe makes four servings. The waffles should be stored in an airtight container in your fridge for no more than five days. They also freeze well and can be stored for three months in your freezer. Be sure to allow the waffles to cool completely before storing them. If you are reheating from the freezer use your toaster so they are nice and crispy.

Veggie Wraps

What you will need:

- ½ cup cherry tomatoes (halved)
- 1 cucumber (cut to thin sticks)
- 6 Kalamata olives (chopped)
- 4 tablespoon feta cheese crumbles
- 2 tablespoons of hummus
- 2 whole-wheat tortilla

Toss everything, except the hummus and tortillas, in a large mixing bowl. Spread a tablespoon of hummus onto a whole-wheat tortilla then add half the tomato mixture over top. Wrap like a burrito.

This recipe makes two servings. You can create the tomato mixture and store it in the refrigerator for up to five days. Assemble the wrap for lunch in the morning or when needed.

Cannellini Bean Salad

What you need:

- 1 tbsp red wine vinegar
- 3 cups cannellini beans, rinsed and drained
- 1 cup cherry tomatoes cut in half
- ½ a red onion, sliced thin
- ¼ cup basil (fresh, torn)

Place all the ingredients into a large salad bowl and toss. Divide the mixture into two servings. Store in the refrigerator for up to seven days. This will make two servings that you will use for lunch during the week.

Quinoa, Vegetable Stir Fry

What you will need:

- 4 tablespoon olive oil
- 2 cups quinoa (cooked according to package instructions)
- 2 garlic cloves (chopped)
- 4 carrots (cut into sticks)
- 2 cups broccoli florets
- ½ cup tomatoes (chopped)
- ½ cup vegetable stock
- 2 tsp tomato puree
- ½ a lemon (juice only)

Cook the garlic in a large frying pan with olive oil for one minute. Add the carrot, broccoli, and leeks and cook for two minutes. Pour in the stock, add the tomatoes, and the tomato puree. Stir, cover, and cook for three minutes. Add the cooked quinoa and stir in the lemon juice.

This will make four servings for dinner. Reserve half a serving for breakfast the next day.

Lentil Shepherd's Pie

For the filling you will need:
- 2 tbsp olive oil
- 4 ½ cup vegetable broth
- 1 ½ cup dry brown lentil
- 1 onion (diced)
- 2 carrots (peeled, diced)
- 2 cups mushrooms (diced)
- 3 garlic cloves (minced)
- ½ cup peas (frozen)
- 2 tbsp tomato paste
- 2 tbsp flour
- 1 tbsp thyme
- ½ tsp sea salt
- ½ tsp black pepper

For the mashed potato topping you will need:
- 2 cups vegetable broth
- 5 large potatoes (peeled, cubed)
- ¼ cup milk
- ¼ tsp sea salt
- ¼ tsp black pepper

To make, boil the potatoes in two cups of vegetable broth and four cups of water for 30 minutes. As the potatoes boil, heat the oil over medium heat in a deep-dish skillet. Add the onions and carrot sand coof for five minutes. Add the mushrooms, stir, and cook for five minutes or until the mushrooms have reduced to half their size. Next, add the garlic and thyme to the skillet. Cook for one minute, stirring frequently. Add the dry lentils, tomato paste, and flour. Stir occasionally and cook for two minutes. Pour in the 4 ½ cups of vegetable broth. Allow the broth to come to a boil, then reduce the heat to medium-low, cover, and simmer for 40 minutes or until the liquids have been absorbed by the lentil. Then add the peas, salt, and black pepper. Stir and set aside.

Once the potatoes are fork-tender, strain them, then return them to the pot. Add the milk, salt, and pepper. Use a potato masher to mash the potatoes until smooth. Set aside and preheat the oven to 400°F (200°C) Once the lentils are done, transfer the mixture to a baking dish and scoop the mashed potatoes over top. Be sure to spread potatoes to the edge of the dish. Bake for 30 minutes or until the top has turned a golden brown. Remove from the oven and cool for 10 minutes before serving.

This recipe will make at least six servings and will be used for one dinner and one lunch option during the week. Leftovers should be stored in an airtight container in your fridge for up to five days. They can also be kept in the freezer for up to three months.

Vegan Sushi Bowl

What you will need:

- 4 cups sushi rice (cooked)
- 1 cup Shiitake mushrooms
- 1 tablespoon coconut aminos
- 1 avocado (sliced)
- 1 cucumber (cut into matchsticks)
- 1 carrot (cut into matchsticks)
- ¼ cup green onion (sliced)
- 4 radish (sliced)

To make the sauce:

- 1 tsp sesame oil
- 1 cup cooked white beans
- 2 tbsp peanut butter
- 1 tsp lime juice

- 2 tbsp rice vinegar
- 2 garlic cloves
- 2 tbsp coconut aminos
- 2 tbsp maple syrup
- ¼ cup water

Heat the oven to 400°F (200°C). In a small bowl toss the mushrooms with coconut aminos. Spread the mushroom onto a baking sheet lined with parchment paper. Bake for 20 minutes or until the edges have started to crisp, remove from the oven. Next, prepare the sauce. Place all the sauce ingredients into a blender and blend until you have a thick but smooth sauce (for a thinner sauce add another tablespoon or two of water). To assemble the bowls, place ¼ to ½ cup of the cooked sushi rice in a bowl. Add some of the cooked mushrooms on top of the rice and then add the cucumber, onions, carrots, avocado, and radish. Drizzle the sauce over top.

This recipe makes four servings and can be used for lunch throughout the week. You can also add crispy tofu to these bowls for extra protein. In the sample menu, this is used as one dinner and one lunch option. Store leftovers in separate containers in your fridge for no more than five days.

Meal Plan

Monday

Breakfast: Tofu scramble and a banana.

Lunch: Cannellini bean salad.

Dinner: Lentil shepherd's pie.

Tuesday

Breakfast: Green Smoothie (blend a cup of water, a cup of kale, two cups of papaya, ½ an avocado, juice from two limes, and one tablespoon of each chia seed and flaxseed).

Lunch: Carrot, orange, and avocado salad: Toss the flesh of one orange, two carrots (shredded), a cup of arugula, and one avocado (seed and peel removed, chopped), with a tablespoon of olive oil and the juice and zest from one orange.

Dinner: Vegan mac and cheese.

Wednesday

Breakfast: Tofu scramble with spinach in a whole wheat wrap.

Lunch: Leftover lentil shepherd's pie.

Dinner: Quinoa, vegetable stir fry.

Thursday

Breakfast: Sweet potato waffles.

Lunch: Veggie wrap.

Dinner: Vegan sushi bowl.

Friday

Breakfast: Tofu scramble with leftover quinoa, vegetable stir fry.

Lunch: Cannellini bean salad.

Dinner: Grilled vegetable kabobs with a side of brown rice and sauteed spinach.

Saturday

Breakfast: Sweet potato waffles.

Lunch: Veggie wrap.

Dinner: Black bean soup.

Sunday

Breakfast: Banana overnight oats (place half a mashed banana, ½ cup soy milk, a teaspoon of cinnamon, 1 / 2 tablespoon each chia seed and flaxseed, and a tablespoon of pure maple syrup in a mason jar. Stir and refrigerator overnight. In the morning, stir again and add a few more slices of banana.

Lunch: Leftover vegan sushi bowl.

Dinner: Loaded sweet potato: Bake sweet potatoes for 45 minutes at 350°F (175°C) then cut them in half. Top with sauteed spinach, red bell peppers, and vidalia onions. Add a scoop of cooked black beans, corn, salsa, and diced avocado.

Chapter 5:

DASH Diet for Menopause

The DASH diet is designed to help treat and prevent hypertension or high blood pressure and emphasizes eating fresh vegetables, fruits, and whole grains. This diet approach eliminates many foods that are known to increase weight and cause other health issues. While the diet is designed to lower cholesterol levels and improve cardiovascular health, it can help you manage your weight during menopause.

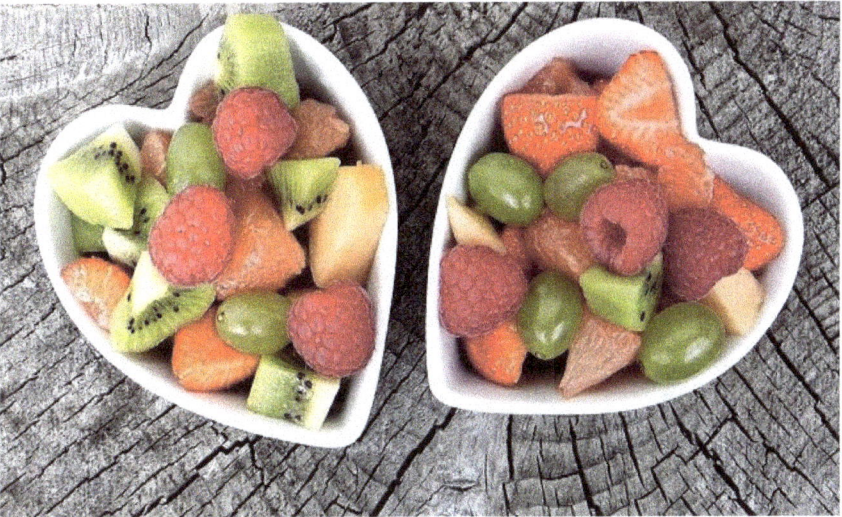

What Is the DASH Diet

The DASH diet is the dietary approach to stop hypertension or high blood pressure. During menopause, women are at a greater risk for heart disease. It has been shown that those who ate a diet high in s and fat are more likely to develop hypertension than those who ate a low-sodium and low-fat diet. This is why the DASH diet emphasizes eating nutrient-rich foods while also being mindful to keep sodium levels in check.

Foods you are encouraged to eat on the DASH diet:

- fruits
- vegetables
- whole grains
- low-fat dairy
- nuts and seeds
- legumes

Foods to limit on the DASH diet include:

- fatty meats including red meat and poultry with the skin left on
- full-fat dairy
- coconut oil and other oils that are solid at room temperature
- added sugar
- sugary foods and drinks like candy, soda, and juice

It is also recommended you cut back on sodium intake. When you first start your goal is to limit sodium to just 2,300 milligrams a day, which equals just a teaspoon of salt a day. Once you have mastered this you continue to limit sodium levels until you reach about 1,500 milligrams a day or less than ¾ a teaspoon.

How the DASH Diet Helps Weight Loss

Though weight loss is not the focus of this diet it is a natural benefit from DASH-ing. Weight loss occurs because the diet provides key health benefits.

High Sodium Intake is Linked to Weight Gain

The average person consumes nearly twice as much sodium than is recommended. Sodium impacts weight because it causes you to retain more water, this excess water is often stored in the blood vessels which puts more pressure on them. When more water is being held in the body, weight gain occurs because you then drink less water as you do not feel thirsty. In addition to this, you will feel more hungry because drinking water can naturally suppress appetite. There is a greater chance that you will overeat more throughout the day causing you to take in more calories, and as a result, you gain weight.

The DASH diet limits high-sodium foods like processed foods, snack foods, and pre-packaged meals. Lower sodium intake to the recommended daily intake of no more than 2,300 milligrams and making it a goal to lower it further to just 1,500 milligrams will significantly impact weight gain. When you lower sodium intake you will begin to first expel all the water weight. What is also important to note is that when you eliminate foods high in sodium and replace them with natural foods like fruits and vegetables you will see even further weight loss.

Lowers Blood Pressure

The dash diet helps keep systolic and diastolic blood pressure in check. Systolic blood pressure is the first number displayed when you get your blood pressure measured. This number represents how much pressure is being exerted on the blood vessels each time your heartbeats. A number below 12o mmHg is considered normal. Diastolic blood pressure is the second number displayed when blood pressure is read. This number measures how much pressure is exerted on the blood vessels in between the heart when the vessels should be more relaxed. A number below 80 mmHg is considered normal or good. Anyone who has a blood pressure reading that is 140/90 or more is considered to have high blood pressure.

One of the most common factors that causes high blood pressure is a diet high in salt, saturated fats, and cholesterol. These are also linked to weight gain. Those who are overweight are more likely to struggle with higher blood pressure as well. High blood pressure is often a precursor to developing heart disease, which is an increased concern for most women during menopause. The DASH diet has been shown to help individuals with high blood pressure lower systolic blood pressure by almost 12 mmHg and lower diastolic levels by over 5 mmHg (Sack et a;., 1999). It has also been shown that lower blood pressure levels occurred even if sodium levels were not reduced and even if the individual did not initially lose weight.

Can Help Lower the Risk of Depression

Many people neglect the link between our mental health and weight. Individuals who are overweight or struggle with their weight are more likely to experience difficulties with their emotions. Emotional eating is a major factor in overeating or binging, as we tend to use food for comfort to temporarily forget about what we are feeling.

This is an important factor to consider as many women going through menopause may struggle with more negative feelings. Shifting hormones can increase the risk of developing depression during menopause. The imbalance of estrogen and progesterone at this time may impact the brain structure and can cause neurotransmitters to malfunction. It is why many women struggle with mood swings and irritability at this time.

When you combine the hormonal shift with the reality that you may be feeling less confident with your changing body or where you are in your life, depression can creep in. These intense feelings of unhappiness and not being interested in things you used to enjoy, increase the possibility that you will reach for more sweet treats and snacks at this time.

Recent studies have shown that the DASH diet can help lower the risk of depression. One such study showed that individuals who closely adhered to the DASH diet instead of a traditional Western diet lowered their risk of developing depression by nearly 11% (Whiteman, 2018). The main factor that is said to help lower this risk is because the DASH diet is low in saturated fats whereas the Western diet is high in these fats and fruits and vegetables are almost absent from meal plans. This same study showed that individuals who consumed a diet high in saturated fats had a much greater risk of suffering from depression and other mental health issues like anxiety.

Is the DASH Diet Right For You?

Women with a history of high blood pressure want to strongly consider the DASH diet. Many who start the DASH find it possible to lower blood pressure in just two weeks. Women who are concerned about their blood pressure will find this diet can ease their worry while also helping them adopt a healthy eating style.

If you are someone who doesn't want to worry about counting calories and instead wants an easy way to lower caloric intake to lose weight, you may find this diet an ideal fit. While it is recommended that you become mindful of what you eat, you shouldn't worry about counting calories to meet a caloric deficit to lose weight. Since the DASH diet encourages eating more fruits and vegetables you will naturally eat fewer calories. This dieting approach has been shown to be a more effective way to lose weight than a traditional low-calorie dieting approach.

If you love to cook you will love this diet. Women who have no problem cooking most or all of their meals tend to be more successful with sticking to the DASH diet. Cooking your meals will help you lower your sodium intake because you will have control over how much salt gets added to what you make. It is not just your meals you need to cook, this goes for making your sauces and condiments, too. Sodium is hidden in nearly all foods you buy from the store, even if it says low-sodium. While it is not a major requirement to limit sodium intake, it is what provides many of the benefits of this diet. If you are more comfortable in the kitchen you will find more pleasure with this diet plan. If you are interested in planning and making most of your meals you struggle to get the results you desire.

How to Get Started

Add an extra serving of fruits and vegetables each day. Most people get one serving of fruits or vegetables a day. To build up to five or more servings start with just adding one more serving at a time. One easy approach to increase fruits and vegetables is to swap out your snack foods. Replace just one snack item with a piece of fruit or raw vegetables sticks.

Don't forget to watch your sodium intake. While your focus will be on eating more wholesome foods it can be easy to ignore lowering sodium consumption. Read food labels carefully. Even low-sodium or reduced-sodium products can still contain high amounts of sodium.

Keep a food journal. Most people do not realize how much they are eating certain foods and how little they eat of others. To help you understand where you are with what you eat and identify what can cause you to struggle with your weight it is best to start recording it all on paper. After two weeks of tracking what you eat, how much you eat, and when, you will spot where you can make changes.

Start to slowly cut back on your sugar consumption. This is another item that many people do not realize how much they are consuming every day. If you drink pop, snack on candy, have a sugary breakfast or indulge in a late-night sweet treat you will struggle with trying to lose weight indefinitely. Sweets are fine every once in a while but many of us consume way more than we want to admit. To help cut back on your sugar intake, find one thing to replace at a time. If you drink a lot of sugary beverages like soda or sweet tea, switch out just one of these drinks a day with a bottle of water. If you enjoy your pastries for breakfast, choose a piece of fruit and yogurt instead of just one day a week. Start with one small change and then add on until you do not even realize that you've gone days with a soda or weeks without a doughnut.

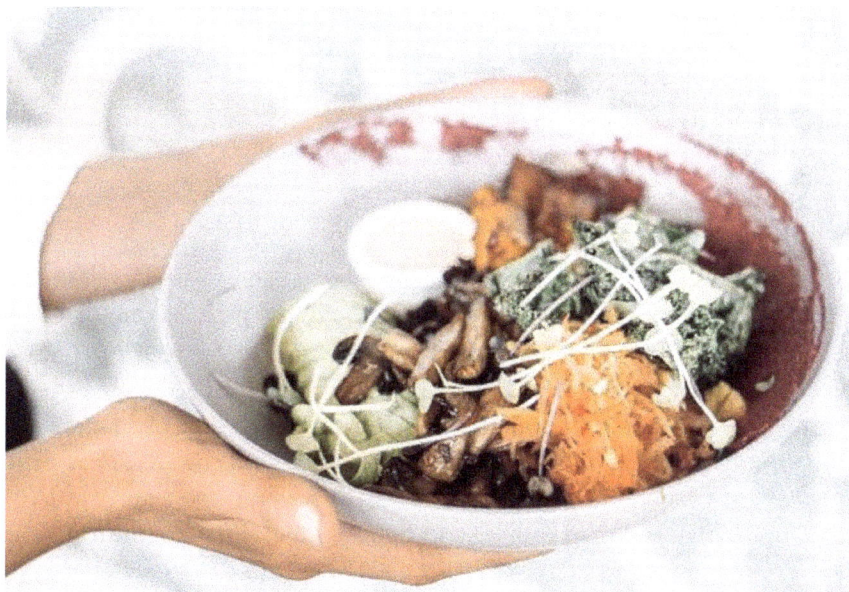

Meal Prep and 7-Day Plan

Recipes and What to Prep

Baked Blueberry Oats

What you will need:

- 3 tbsp melted coconut oil (divided)
- ⅓ cup pure maple syrup
- 2 cup old-fashioned oats
- 1 ¾ cup almond milk

- 2 flax eggs (stir 2 tbsp ground flaxseed with 6 tbsp water and let sit for 5 minutes)
- ⅔ cup chopped pecans
- 2 ½ cups blueberries
- 1 tsp baking powder
- ¼ tsp ground nutmeg
- 2 tsp cinnamon
- 2 tsp pure vanilla extract
- ¼ tsp sea salt

Heat the oven to 375°F (190°C) and grease a 9x9-inch baking dish, **set aside.** Line a baking sheet with parchment paper and spread the pecans across in a single layer. Bake for five minutes, remove the oven, cool slightly, then transfer to a mixing bowl of medium size. Add the oats, cinnamon, nutmeg, baking powder, and salt in with the pecans. Stir to combine and set to the side. Take a small mixing bowl and beat the eggs, milk, maple syrup, vanilla, and half of the melted coconut oil. Set aside.

Add half the blueberries to the bottom of the baking dish, then top with the oat mixture. Pour the milk and egg mixture over the oats and give the dish a little shake so the milk seeps through the oats. Arrange the remaining blueberries over top and bake for 45 minutes. Once the oats have turned a deep golden brown, remove them from the oven, and drizzle the remaining melted coconut oil over top.

This recipe makes six servings. You can use it as a breakfast option or an after-dinner snack topped with a quarter cup of Greek yogurt. Keep any leftovers in your refrigerator for five days.

Chickpea Curry

What you will need:

- 3 tbsp olive oil
- 2 15-ounce cans of chickpeas (drained and rinsed)
- ¼ cup vegetable stock

- 2 ¼ cups diced tomatoes
- 1 yellow onion (chopped)
- 4 garlic cloves
- 1 2-inch piece of ginger (chopped)
- 2 tsp ground coriander
- 2 tsp ground cumin
- 1 tsp ground turmeric
- 2 tsp garam masala
- ¼ tsp sea salt

Place the garlic, ginger, and onions into a processorocess and pulse until finely chopped, set aside. Add the oil to a large saucepan and warm it over medium-high heat, then add the onion mixture to the pan. Cook for five minutes and stir occasionally. Add the coriander, cumin, and turmeric and cook for another two minutes. Place the tomatoes and vegetable stock into the food processor and pulse until finely chopped then add to the pan with the onions. Bring to a boil, then lower heat to medium and simmer for five minutes. Add the chickpeas, garam masala, and salt and simmer for another five minutes, stir occasionally.

This recipe will make six servings. Keep the leftovers in your fridge for no more than a week.

Fruit Kabobs

What you will need:

- 4 pineapple chunks (½-inch piece)
- 2 strawberries
- 1 kiwi (quartered, the skin is edible and can be left on for more nutrients)
- 1 banana (1/2 -inch pieces)
- 4 grapes
- 1 tsp lime juice
- 1 tsp lime zest

- 6 oz Greek yogurt
- 1 tbsp honey

Mix the yogurt, honey, lime juice, and lime zest in a small bowl. Chill in the fridge until you are ready to serve. You will need four wooden skewers for the kabobs. Take a skewer and place one piece of fruit on each. Serve with the yogurt mixture.

This recipe will make two servings (2 skewers per serving). You can make a huge batch of these ahead of time (add the banana only when you are ready to serve to prevent browning) and use them for snacks throughout the week.

Tomato and Watermelon Salad

What you will need:
- 1 tbsp extra virgin olive oil
- 1 tbsp red wine vinegar
- ½ cup tomatoes (chopped)
- 3 cups watermelon (cubed)
- ½ cup feta cheese crumbles
- 1 tbsp fresh mint (chopped)

Place all the ingredients into a large salad bowl. Toss so everything is nicely coated with the oil and vinegar.

This recipe will make two servings. It can be used for lunch but in the meal plan sample, it is used for a snack option. You can store this salad in the refrigerator for up to three days.

Raspberry Cocoa Chia Seed Pudding

What you will need:
- 1 cup almond milk
- 1 cup fresh raspberries

- 4 tbsp chia seed
- 1 tbsp pure maple syrup
- 1 tsp cocoa powder (unsweetened)
- ½ tsp pure vanilla extract
- 2 tbsp sliced almonds

In a small bowl, stir the almond milk, chia seeds, syrup, cocoa, and vanilla. Cover and chill for at least 8 hours and up to 3 days. To serve, divide the mixture in half and top with half the raspberries and half the almond slice.

This recipe makes two servings, It can be used as a breakfast option or snack.

Meal Plan

Monday

Breakfast: Baked blueberry oats.

Snack: Greek yogurt and banana parfait topped with two tablespoons of chopped walnuts.

Lunch: Two pieces of whole-grain toast topped with cottage cheese and peach slices.

Snack: Tomato and watermelon salad.

Dinner: Herb crusted salmon served with roast small potatoes and brussel sprouts.

Tuesday

Breakfast: Two eggs on whole-wheat toast topped with tomatoes and spinach.

Snack: Blueberry cranberry smoothie (blend half a frozen banana, ½ cup frozen blueberries, ½ cup frozen cranberries, and a cup of Greek yogurt).

Lunch: Spinach, tomato, and swiss quesadillas (use whole wheat tortilla) topped with guacamole and salsa.

Snack: Fruit Kabobs.

Dinner: Chickpea curry.

Wednesday

Breakfast: Baked blueberry oats.

Snack: Tomato and watermelon salad.

Lunch: Veggie wrap made with ¼ cup cherry tomatoes (halved), ½ a cucumber (cut to thin sticks), a fourth of a red bell pepper (cut into stripes), and a tablespoon of hummus wrapped in a whole-wheat tortilla. Serve with half a cup of Greek yogurt and mixed berries.

Snack: Fruit kabobs.

Dinner: Whole-wheat pasta with sauteed spinach and mushroom and a pesto sauce.

Thursday

Breakfast: Baked blueberry oats.

Snack: Half a cup of Greek yogurt with ½ cup fresh raspberries, 1 tablespoon almond slices and drizzled with a teaspoon of pure maple syrup.

Lunch: Grilled chicken with tomato, cucumber, onions, and lettuce in a whole-wheat pita drizzle with tzatziki sauce.

Snack: Raspberry cocoa chia seed pudding.

Dinner: Gnocchi with a tomato basil sauce and steamed vegetables on the side.

Friday

Breakfast: Avocado toast sprinkled with hemp seed and flaxseed, along with a piece of fruit.

Snack: Fruit kabobs.

Lunch: Leftover chickpea curry.

Snack: Raspberry cocoa chia seed pudding.

Dinner: Grilled chicken and roasted summer squash over spinach with a lemon vinaigrette.

Saturday

Breakfast: Mushroom, spinach, and tomato omelet.

Snack: Mix berries and ¼ cup Greek yogurt.

Lunch: Two hard-boiled eggs with 2 cups spinach, ¼ cup feta cheese, 1.2 cup diced cucumbers, and 1.2 cups cherry tomatoes. Drizzle with a red wine vinaigrette.

Snack: Banana slices and nut butter on whole-wheat toast.

Dinner: Roasted vegetables over brown rice.

Sunday

Breakfast: Black bean burrito and a side of mixed fruit.

Snack: Green smoothie: Blend ½ cup swiss chard, ½ cup kale, an apple and a pear (seed and core removed), ½ cup blueberries, ¼ cup goji berries, 10 cashews, 2 tablespoons raw cacao, 2 tablespoons flaxseed, 1 cup water, and ½ cup almond milk.

Lunch: Leftover chickpea curry.

Snack: Fruit kabobs.

Dinner: Eggplant parmesan.

Chapter 6:

Food to Focus On

The quality of the food you eat matters more as you get older. During menopause, there are foods you want to add to your diet to help alleviate and manage symptoms of menopause while also helping you lose weight. These foods can help you feel more comfortable and confident without negatively influencing your weight loss goals.

Foods to Help with Weight Loss and Weight Management

What you eat and how much you eat are equally important when it comes to keeping weight off during menopause. If you are trying to lose weight during this time it is essential that you consume a caloric deficit (you are eating fewer calories than your body is burning) is often the go-to method for weight loss. This approach can backfire during menopause when your resting metabolism is slower, so you are not burning as many calories when you are not physically active.

With a slower resting metabolism when you consume fewer calories it can make losing weight even harder. You get stuck in a vicious cycle because during menopause you also lose muscles mass which is what helps burn calories even at rest. Being mindful of your caloric intake is one way to help minimize weight gain, but there are a few other tricks to know that can help keep your weight in check.

While you want to consume the right number of calories it is also important to be mindful of the foods you are eating. Eating foods that are nutrient-rich while also having a lower number of calories is the most effective approach to losing weight. This does not mean you should eat other nutrient-rich foods that may be high in calories. Below you will find a food list to help you with your meal planning for a well-balanced diet that will promote weight loss.

High Fiber Foods

You should be aiming to get between 20 to 25 grams of fiber into your diet daily. High fiber foods include:

- beans and lentils (kidney beans, split peas, black beans, and chickpeas have the highest fiber content)
- artichoke
- brussels sprouts

- broccoli
- kale
- avocado
- quinoa
- oats
- apples
- berries
- pears
- chia seeds
- pistachios
- sunflower seeds
- almonds

Consume these high-fiber foods first with your meals. This will help keep you feeling full for longer. Fiber-rich foods also help clear the digestive tract.

Complex Carbs

Complex carbs such as lentils, beans, and whole grains are broken down and turned into glucose to fuel the body. These carbs are processed more slowly than simple carbs. Complex carbs also help combat abdominal fat from building up.

One thing to keep in mind about these different carbs; many fruits are considered simple carbs because the sugars in them are broken down quickly. Unlike refined sugar sources, fruits contain a high amount of fiber, too. Fiber helps slow down digestion and therefore does not release the glucose into the body as rapidly as it would from table sugar, candy, soda, and other refined sugar items.

Eat Enough Protein

Protein impacts your weight in a few key ways during menopausal years. It is essential to maintain healthy bone density and muscle mass.

You also need it to keep your metabolism up and will keep the immune system functioning properly. Many of our body's functions rely on various components of protein to function properly, this includes hormone production. When you eat lean protein you will also feel satisfied and stay full for longer.

Starting your day off with eggs can help boost your weight loss efforts during menopause. One study showed that individuals who ate a breakfast that included eggs as opposed to one that only included whole grains or carbohydrates saw a 61 percent reduction in their body mass index and lost 65 percent more weight (Wal et al., 2008).

Water

Start each meal with a glass of water. Try to sip on water in between meals instead of automatically reaching for a snack. Most times we mix up our hunger cues and thirst cues as the body interprets both the same way. When you are feeling hungry you may just need a little extra hydration. Sip on some water and then wait to see if your hunger diminishes.

Foods That Help with Hormonal Balance

Everything we eat impacts our health; this can be in a positive or negative way. The nutrients food provides us helps maintain proper hormone production and distribution. Eating a well-balanced diet can allow the body to keep hormones in check, but during menopause, there are certain foods that you want to consume more of to combat the effects of changing hormone levels.

Organic Grass-Fed Lean Protein

Animal meat provides us with essential amino acids. These amino acids are necessary for maintaining muscle mass, bone density, and are the building blocks for cells and tissues in the body. There are 20 amino acids the body needs to properly function, many of which the body produces on its own. Other amino acids are essential to help the body better use the ones it makes naturally. For example; the body naturally produces the amino acid Carnitine. Carnitine keeps the liver, kidneys, brain, heart, and skeletal muscles strong and functioning properly. Carnitine is also needed when turning fat into energy. To ensure carnitine is properly used and distributed throughout the body, it needs help from another amino acid Lysine. While the body naturally produces Creatine, Lysine can only be obtained by the foods we eat, especially lean protein.

You should look to add a variety of lean meats to your diet as you age, including poultry, eggs, and red meats. How much protein you need depends on your weight. Women should aim to consume half their body weight in grams of protein daily. For example, if you weigh 160 pounds you want to consume 80 grams of protein daily, which is just under three ounces. Also, include wild-caught fish which provides you with omega-3 fatty acids which are vital for brain health. Those who are choosing to stick with a vegan or vegetarian diet can still get many of the amino acids they need from plant-based sources, but it is important that you consult with your doctor to ensure you are getting enough of each amino acid. There are supplements available to reduce the risk of missing out on these key nutrients.

Another thing to consider when planning your grocery list; you want quality lean proteins. Buying organic and grass-fed products minimizes consuming unwanted chemicals. Many factory-raised animals are given a diet filled with hormones. These hormones are then absorbed by you when you consume them which can make keeping your hormones in balance more challenging.

Healthy Fats

Healthy fats are unsaturated, monounsaturated, or polyunsaturated fats. Avocados are especially good at balancing hormones because they are rich in monounsaturated fatty acids, potassium, vitamin E, B vitamin, folic acid, magnesium, and fiber. Try adding half an avocado a day to your diet for the best benefits.

Green Tea

Green tea has many powerful antioxidants that have a positive impact on overall health, especially cardiovascular health. Menopausal women benefit even further from drinking green tea because of its catechins polyphenols and epigallocatechin gallate (EGCg). These are specific antioxidants that help clear free radicals from the body and improve cholesterol levels. This can result in better hormonal balance throughout the body.

Vegetables

Cruciferous vegetables like broccoli, brussels sprouts, and cauliflower release a powerful phytochemical (3-carbinol) that helps with liver function. The liver helps produce and distribute various hormones like insulin. Eating a wide variety of vegetables from dark leafy greens to colorful carrots and bell peppers provides you with essential nutrients and vitamins. Consuming vegetables not only will help maintain better overall help but will ensure the body is getting what it needs to minimize hormonal imbalance. Your goal should be to eat five to seven servings of vegetables a day. Each serving should be around a cup of cooked, steamed, or raw vegetables.

Flaxseed and Soybeans

Flaxseed and soybeans contain phytoestrogens to help regulate estrogen levels slightly. Soy contains isoflavones that bind estrogen receptors in the body. Flaxseeds contain lignans which have estrogenic effects when consumed. Flaxseeds can be found in whole seeds or ground. They can be added to many dishes from breakfast oats, smoothies, and soups. When mixed with water, ground flax can be used in baking and other recipes as an egg replacement.

Herbs and Spices

Not only is it a great idea to incorporate more herbs and spices into your meals for different flavors they can help fight off inflammation. The anti-inflammatory components allow the body to keep hormone levels balanced. Herbs and spices can be used in many ways from fresh, dried, whole seeds, and ground. Some of the most powerful herbs and spices to consume more of include turmeric, ginger, and garlic.

Magnesium-Rich Foods

Magnesium is essential for helping the body regulate blood sugar and insulin levels. It can also help with regulating the nervous system, nutrient absorption, and distributing hormones. Some of the best food sources that are high in magnesium include spinach, kale, avocado, chickpeas, soybeans, tofu, brazilian nuts, almonds, pumpkin seed, sunflower seed, quinoa.

Foods to Avoid

Processed food, caffeine, and fatty meats. Processed foods lack nutrients which can make it harder for the body to produce the hormones it needs. Caffeine increases the stress hormone cortisol which not only can cause you to overeat, it can impact many other systems in the body such as the sleep cycle. Fatty meat that is high in saturated fats decreases serotonin levels, which is the body's feel-good hormone. If you are struggling with frequent mood swings, increased anger, or irritability you may want to check in with how much fatty meats like bacon you are consuming. This could be the cause of your unpredictable mood.

Foods to Combat Hot Flashes

Hot flashes can strike out of nowhere and leave you feeling uncomfortable and slightly embarrassed. Have you ever had a sudden rush of fire hit you standing in line at the grocery store? It's not pleasant or enjoyable. One of the most common complaints of women going through menopause is the uncontrollable hot flashes they experience. With the foods listed below, you will learn that you can have better control of your body temperature. With these foods, you can reduce the frequency and even eliminate hot flashes from occurring.

Soy

Soy is the number one food that has been shown to help reduce and even eliminate hot flashes in menopausal women. Soy has similar binding agents as estrogen. When you consume soy you can block receptors in the body that cause your temperature to rise and lead to hot flashes. The best sources of soy are tofu and tempeh. You can also drink soy milk, eat edamame as a snack, or try adding some miso to your dishes.

Low Glycemic Index Foods

There has been a connection between body temperature and the release of insulin which is produced to carry glucose to cells throughout the body. When insulin levels are high body temperature increases. Low glycemic foods do not cause a high or consistent spike in insulin levels. This means we won't produce as much heat. Including more low glycemic index foods can help keep hot flashes at a minimum during the day and through the evening.

Low glycemic foods to incorporate into your diet include:

- non-starchy vegetables (especially eggplant, carrots, peppers, and broccoli)
- fruits (grapefruit, apricots, apples, and strawberries)
- legumes and beans (especially chickpeas, kidney beans, and black beans)
- yogurt
- nuts and seed (walnuts, macadamia, chia, and flax)
- oats
- barley

Cooling Foods

Cooling foods have been used in Chinese medicine to help lower body temperature. What is great about these foods is that they also provide plenty of nutrients to keep you healthy during and after menopause. Some of the best known cooling foods to try include:

- banana
- spinach
- broccoli
- eggs
- apples
- cold water

Foods to Avoid

There are several foods that you will want to avoid during menopause as these are known to make hot flashes worse. Alcohol, caffeine, and of course spicy foods, will all increase the intensity and frequency of hot flashes. It is best to avoid these or enjoy them only occasionally during menopause.

Foods for Better Sleep

Sleep and diet have a complex relationship. If you are not eating a well-balanced diet chances are you are struggling with sleep issues. If you are having sleep issues it is more likely that you are going to make poor food choices. During menopause, it is more common for women to have difficulty sleeping due to hot flashes, extra stress and anxiety, and disruption to hormone production. There are foods you can incorporate into your diet to improve your quality and duration of sleep.

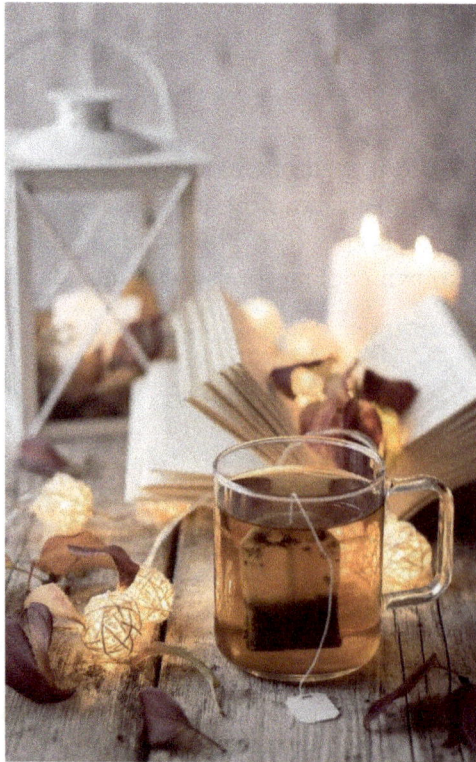

Nuts and Seeds

Almonds specifically can help promote a good night's sleep. Almonds help combat inflammation which can disrupt sleep. They also contain melatonin, which is the body's natural sleep hormone. They also provide you with magnesium which helps lower cortisol (stress hormone) levels in the body. Walnuts are another nut that contains magnesium, melatonin, and serotonin.

Milk

Drinking warm milk before bed is looked at as an old-school sleep remedy. Maybe your grandparents warmed you up with a glass of milk before bed when you stayed with them or maybe your mom did the same for you when you were younger. Drinking warm milk improves sleep because it contains tryptophan, calcium, melatonin, and vitamin D. When these components are combined with the comfort you may get from the memories of drinking this beverage before bed when you were younger, you have the perfect recipe for a good night's sleep. Low-fat milk also promotes better sleep. Additionally, a warm cup of milk can help relax the body much in the same way a warm cup of tea can so you feel ready for sleep.

Vegetables

Lettuce, tomatoes, carrots, and pumpkin may all help you get a better night's sleep. Garden and wild lettuce contain lactucarium which has sedative properties. Tomatoes are high in phytonutrient lycopene which has been shown to help you stay asleep. It is best to eat the tomatoes warm and simmered in a little oil or fat so the lycopene can be more easily absorbed by the body. Carrots and pumpkins contain carotenoids which can improve sleep.

Dark leafy greens can also help combat the effects of poor sleeping habits. These vegetables are an excellent source of iron which has been shown to protect against sleep disorders like restless leg syndrome.

Legumes and Beans

Legumes and beans contain high amounts of B-vitamins (B6, B12, and folic acid). These vitamins are essential for regulating the body's natural sleep-wake cycle. They are also associated with an increase in serotonin which will help you feel relaxed and ready for sleep. You can choose any variety of legumes and beans to feel the benefits. Alfalfa, peas, soy, and peanuts are all part of the bean and legume family that provide you with plenty of B vitamins for better sleep.

Whole Grains

Brown rice, whole-wheat bread or pasta, and quinoa contain high amounts of magnesium, calcium, and potassium. Potassium specifically is a natural muscle relaxant that can help you drift off to sleep. You want to avoid processed grains like white flour, white bread or pasta, and white rice, as these will cause insulin levels to spike and will contribute to feeling restless.

Tryptophan

Tryptophan is an amino acid that can increase melatonin production. Melatonin is the body's sleep hormone. Turkey is one of the most well-known sleep boosters because it contains tryptophan. This is why so many people are ready for a nap after eating Thanksgiving dinner. Tryptophan is also found in chicken breast and tart cherry juice. For tryptophan to work is sleeping magic, however, it needs to be consumed with a small amount of carbohydrates so that it can be carried over the brain barrier. Try eating a small portion of brown rice or quinoa with chicken or turkey a few hours before bed to help you fall asleep faster.

Other Foods to Eat Before Bed

Chamomile tea is also a go-to beverage right before bed. Chamomile contains apigenin which is an antioxidant that can help increase tiredness. It has also been shown to help combat insomnia.

Kiwi Fruit has also been studied and proven to help promote a better night's sleep. In one study individuals who consumed kiwi an hour before bed were able to fall asleep faster than individuals who did not (Elliott, 2020). Kiwi's ability to help you fall asleep is linked to its effect on serotonin which is the brains' sleep cycle chemical.

Tart cherry juice also contains a significant amount of melatonin. Women who struggle to fall asleep or stay asleep may find improvement in their sleep by drinking a small amount of tart cherry juice before bed.

Foods to Avoid

Avoid alcohol and caffeine if you are struggling to fall asleep or stay asleep through the night. These will increase cortisol levels (stress hormone) which will make it harder to sleep. Spicy foods or foods that can cause heartburn should also be avoided.

You should also try to avoid skipping meals throughout the day as this can throw off the balance of certain hormones that can promote sleep. It is also important to keep yourself hydrated as dehydration can cause you to be sleepless.

Chapter 7:

Dieting Tips

There are a lot of poor dieting tips that may sound good at first but are not going to help you feel your best. In this chapter, we will discuss some bad dieting tips you might get as you get older and which tips you should follow.

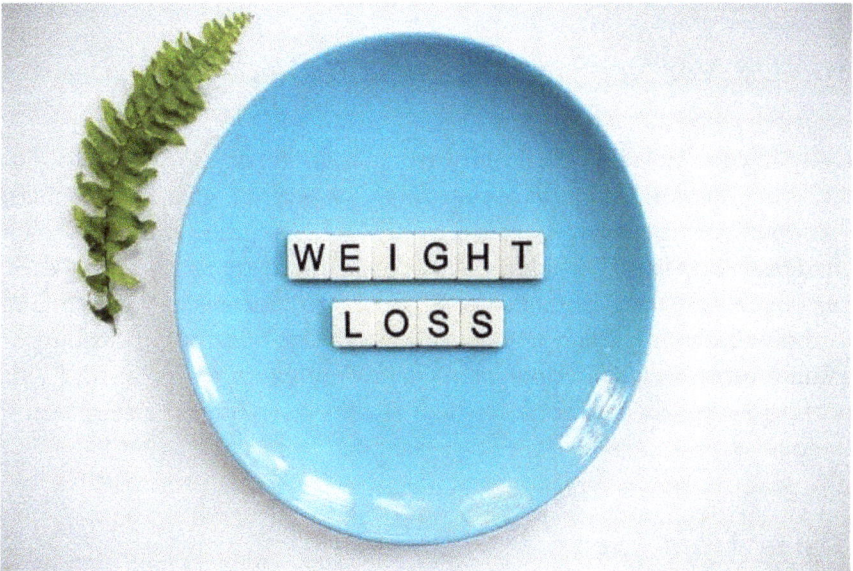

Dieting Tips You Might Believe (but shouldn't follow)

You may have been told a few things that sound legitimate when it comes to getting through menopause. While these things may sound reasonable, they often do not take into consideration all that is changing with your body. Below are a few misconceptions about what you should or shouldn't do as you enter menopause and beyond. We will debunk these suggestions and let you know what you should consider instead.

You Do Not Need to Change Your Diet

Even if you stick to a fairly healthy diet, some of the foods you are including in your diet may contribute to weight gain and increase menopause symptoms. Because your body is going through many changes it is essential to address your diet. There are foods you need to cut back on and others you need to increase your intake. Carbohydrates, for example, even the healthier ones can contribute to gaining more weight during menopause. You want to reconsider your portion sizes when it comes to carbs and how often you are eating them.

Try to Avoid Exercise

Many women feel that exercise will only increase their risk of injury because of the decrease in bone density. There is also the limiting belief that many women adopt as they get older that they are "just too old" to get fit. This is anything but the truth. Exercise is essential for maintaining your strength among other things. You do not need to do workouts that are hard on the joints. Many types of exercise will get your heart rate up which will lead to burning more calories while also helping you build lean muscle.

It is Ok to Nap During the Day

When you struggle to get enough sleep in the evening it is tempting to squeeze in some extra sleep during the day. While sometimes taking a nap during the day may be necessary, midday snoozing will only make it more difficult to get the quality and quantity of sleep you need in the evening hours. If you must nap during the day limit it to no more than an hour, ideally you want to stick to a short power nap of only 20 minutes. Sleeping for long during the day is going to cut into your sleeping hours in the evening.

You are Going Through Menopause

Menopause can cause your body to go through a number of changes other serious health issues can arise. While, yes, you will experience a number of symptoms because of menopause you should not brush everything off as menopausal symptoms. If you are struggling with sleep or weight loss especially if you have changed your diet and increased your exercise consider talking to your doctor. They can help you identify other factors that might be causing you issues.

Additionally, do not become a victim of letting menopause be an excuse for sticking with poor habits that are not serving you. Losing weight, feeling confident about yourself, and improving your health can all be accomplished despite going through menopause. It can feel like a struggle at times when you feel like your body is fighting against you but rest assured, menopause only last for a brief time and after that, you will want to be feeling your best!

Dieting Tips to Follow

While it is easy to discuss what you should or should not eat during menopause another important element is your relationship with food. If you look at food as an enemy you will struggle with making them better for your choices. If you tell yourself you can't eat something you will feel guilty when you indulge in foods that may not be so great for you. Addressing eating habits is just as important as choosing the most nutritious foods to consume.

Mindful eating and intuitive eating are two approaches to consider to help build a better relationship around food. With these approaches, you learn to slow down and get in tune with how your body feels before, during, and after you eat. This will allow you to identify foods that can trigger menopause symptoms like hot flashes, lower mood, difficulty sleeping along with other discomforts like feeling bloated and having excess gas.

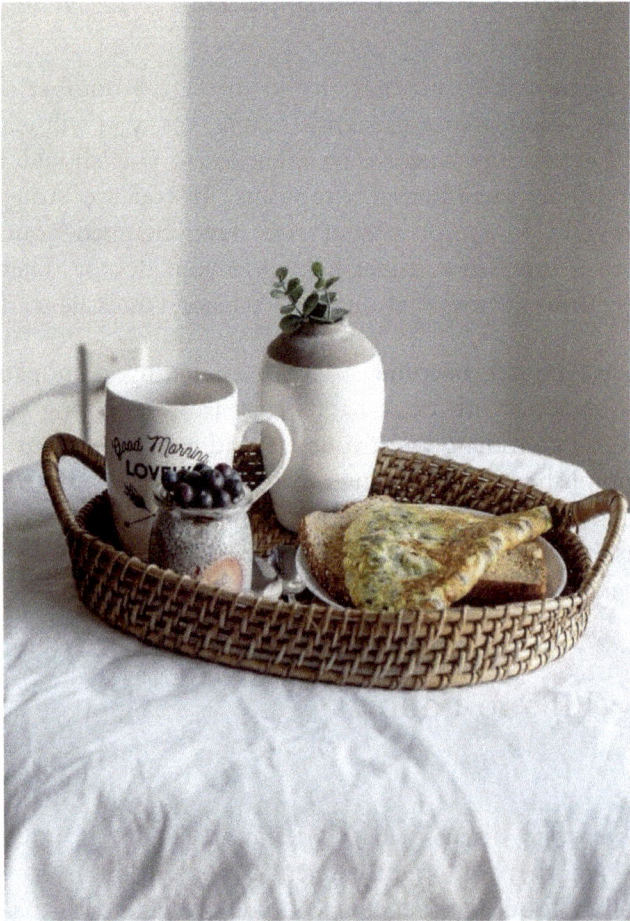

Mindful Eating

Mindfulness eating breaks a meditative twist to your meals. We often rush through what we eat without taking a moment to pause and enjoy what we eat. Even during menopause your schedule is probably packed with things to do and grabbing something quick and easy to eat in the car or before your next meeting has probably become the norm. Rushing through meals can cause us to overeat and choose foods that are not the best for us. Instead, mindfulness eating gives us an opportunity to slow down. With mindfulness eating, we tune into our senses as we eat. We notice the smell, texture, and taste of our food. We let certain foods bring back fond memories of our childhood or we take a moment to appreciate the company we have at that time.

Mindfulness eating can extend through the whole process of preparing our meals as well. We can be more mindful as we shop for the foods to include in our meals, we can be more mindful as we prepare and cook our meals. This is a non-judgemental act. We do not beat ourselves up for purchasing something that might not be too great for us and we do not over congratulate ourselves when we only choose healthy foods. Instead, we take note of how we feel in the moment and move on to the next moment.

Intuitive Eating

Intuitive eating is similar to mindful eating but takes things a little deeper by guiding you to build a healthy relationship with food by listening to your body's natural cues. Intuitive eating is a process where you honor your body. When you are hungry, eat. If you are full, you stop eating. When you crave something you allow yourself to have it. It is also a practice where you show your body respect daily by choosing to fuel it with nutritious foods. Intuitive eating uses a framework of 10 principles that do not focus on what you eat or what you shouldn't eat. Instead, these principles provide a new perspective on how to approach food so that you are comfortable eating foods that make you feel good. They also provide a structure to build additional health habits.

The 10 principles of intuitive eating include:

1. Reject the diet mindset.

The diet mindset fills you with false hope of losing weight quickly and that you will keep the weight off. It is this idea that if you drastically change what you eat you will see fast results. It does not address healthy eating habits that promote weight management for the long term. We have discussed a few diet plan options in this book that can lead to weight loss. The main focus is that these are sustainable ways of eating. If you continue to think the next fad diet is the only way you will lose weight, you will continue to fall victim to a vicious cycle. You may lose weight but since the faded diet is not sustainable the weight will come back. Rejecting the diet mindset means rejecting the idea that a quick-fix diet plan is going to help you maintain a healthy weight for the long term.

2. Honor your hunger cues.

This principle is simple to follow. When you feel hungry, eat. So often we tend to ignore our hunger cues, especially when trying to lose weight. What ends up happening is we go for a long period of time feeling hunger that by the time we do sit down to eat we overeat which only leads to feeling guilty for not having more self-control.

3. Food is neither good nor bad.

When trying to lose weight it is common for people to split foods into good or bad. You try to stick with the good foods and tell yourself you can't have the bad foods. Most people who are told not to do something end up having a greater desire to do what they shouldn't, and this is true with food. Not allowing yourself to eat a certain food because it is considered bad for you will more often than not lead to overindulging in that food. Instead, food should be looked at for what it is; a means to fuel your body. To provide it with nutrients and vitamins that it needs.

4. You are not good or bad because of your food choices.

You are neither good nor bad because of your food choices. How often have you told yourself that you are horrible for eating that chocolate cake, or how good you were today because you stuck to a healthy eating plan and ate below your calorie goals? When we tell ourselves we are good or bad for what we eat we tend to be overly critical. The negative talk this often leads to will decrease your motivation for eating the foods that promote better health.

5. Enjoy your food.

This aligns with mindfulness eating but takes it a step further. When you fully enjoy your food you feel satisfied and will gain more pleasure from what you eat. This extends beyond what is on your plate. Where you eat, the environment around you should add to these feelings of satisfaction. Think about it, how much do you fully enjoy your meals when you are in an overcrowded place with terrible lighting and an odd odor? You can create an atmosphere around you that will lead to gaining more pleasure from what you eat, whether it is a salad or an ice cream sundae. When you are in the right environment you can bring more awareness to what you are eating and will better decide how much is enough to feel satiated.

6. Honor your fullness.

Just as you want to honor your hunger cues you also want to honor the cues your body gives you when you are full. Many people were brought up being told they needed to clear their plate and they carry this through their adult years. They force themselves to continue eating even when they are completely stuffed and taking another bite often makes them feel sick. Build trust with your body and respect it by stopping when it says it has had enough. Make it a habit to pause during your meal to check in with your hunger. Ask yourself how much you are enjoying what you are eating or how good it tastes. The more we eat the less satisfaction we begin to gain from the flavor of our food. Also, ask yourself how hungry you still are. If you are beginning to feel full it is time to stop eating.

7. Food is not meant to feed your emotions.

Many of us, unintentionally, turn to food for comfort. Some of us have been taught to do this from a young age. How many of you were offered ice cream when dealing with a breakup as a child or after a big test got rewarded with a plate of freshly baked cookies? As we have grown, the emotional connection we have with food has only strengthened. On top of this, if you have constantly jumped from diet to diet, you may struggle with feeling like you have control over your eating habits. This lack of control can lead to emotional eating. We need to find more gentle and effective ways to address our emotions that do not involve food. Turning to food for comfort or to ignore what we feel will not fix the problem and more often causes us to feel even worse.

8. Respect your body.

The big problem with dieting and the mindset that comes along with it is that it often causes us to have an unrealistic expectation of how our body is supposed to look. We are all created to be different and unique, thinking you need to fit into a smaller size or look a certain way will lead to disappointment and discomfort. Instead, respect the body you have and what it can do. When we love our body we will be less critical of how we look. This will then allow us to focus on all that we can do. Appreciate what your body has done for you and what it will continue to do for you. When you adopt this mindset you will begin to be more mindful of taking care of your body and loving it in the best way.

9. Feel your workouts.

Working out should not be just about how many calories you burn. Looking at exercising as something you have to do to get in shape and lose weight is not the best way to motivate yourself to work out. Exercising should be something you enjoy because of how it makes you feel. If you struggle to stick with an exercise routine, try focusing on how energized you feel, how it builds your confidence or lifts your mood for the rest of the day. Shifting your focus to how you feel during and after your workout will serve as a greater motivation and will help you stick with an exercise routine.

10. Honor your health.

What you eat and how often you get moving should be about your overall health. You do not have to eat perfectly all the time to be healthy. Having one dessert is not going to cause you to become overweight, just like having one salad is not going to cause you to lose a drastic amount of weight. What you eat most of the time and what you do most days will have the greatest impact on your health. You want to enjoy your food while also being mindful of your health but this does not mean you have to deprive yourself of foods you enjoy. When it comes to losing weight there should be more focus on making progress, not eating perfectly. If you put in the effort to continuously make the best choice for yourself, then you are going in the right direction.

Chapter 8:

Get Yourself Moving

Exercise is vital for staying healthy after 40. While changing what you eat can help jumpstart weight loss, exercise will streamline your efforts so you see more weight loss in a short time. Learn what exercises are best during menopause and how to make physical activity a healthy habit for life.

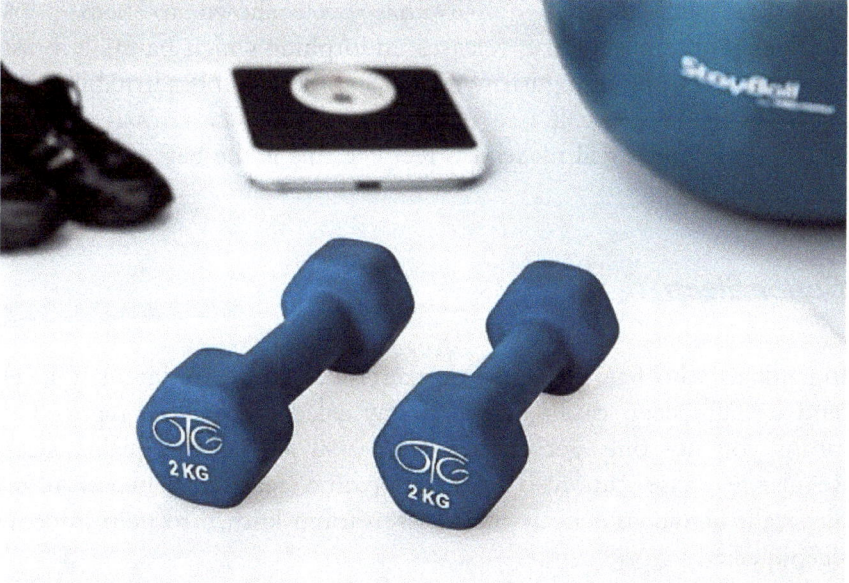

How Exercise Will Help You Through Menopause

Exercise can help further alleviate the symptoms of menopause. While most people look at exercise as another way to help them lose weight it has a much wider-reaching impact on various aspects of your health.

Better Mood

During menopause, many women struggle to feel good about themselves and physical activity has been shown to help boost confidence. Exercising also releases endorphins which naturally boost your mood. Fitting in regular workouts can help combat irritability and mood swings because it is a natural way to reduce stress. All these benefits combined will make you feel like this is the best time of your life.

Better Sleep

Individuals who fit a few days or exercise at moderate intensity levels tend to fall asleep easier and also stay asleep the whole night. This means you not only get enough sleep you are getting quality sleep. Regular exercise can also reduce daytime fatigue. When you are physically active your body releases serotonin known to help improve sleep quality.

Improve Flexibility, Mobility, and Balance

More flexibility, ease of mobility, and improved balance will allow you to move your body with more ease during menopause. This also lowers the risk of age-related injuries that are common as we get older. As we get older we may struggle more with balance which can cause us to trip and fall more often. When these accidental falls are combined with lower bone density there is a greater risk for serious injuries. Breaking or spraining an ankle, wrist, or even hip will lead to limited physical activity, which in turn, will often result in more weight gain.

Keep Hormones In Check

Exercising for 30 minutes a day and getting the heart pumping can help increase estrogen levels. This boost in estrogen can help alleviate many symptoms of menopause. Exercising also increases dopamine levels. Dopamine is a hormone that can help lower stress and anxiety.

Reduce the Risk of Osteoporosis

Working out will improve bone density which is often lost during menopause. Weight training and strength training exercises will allow you to maintain strong bones which lowers the risk of osteoporosis.

Heart Health

The decrease in estrogen levels during menopause increases the risk of heart disease. Lower levels of estrogen have been linked to an increase in bad cholesterol levels. Exercise is one of the best natural ways to keep your heart healthy.

Types of Exercise for Weight Loss

- Yoga. Yoga is ideal for improving range of motion and flexibility. It is also effective to combat stress and helps keep the mind focused and sharp. You can incorporate yoga throughout your day. Performing an easy 10-minute yoga routine in the morning helps stretch the muscle and can even help stimulate the digestive tract. If yoga is not your thing, simply taking 5 to 10 minutes to stretch periodically throughout the day can improve muscle and tendon mobility.

- Tai chi. This is a low-impact meditative type of exercise. While tai chi may look like very slow-moving karate it has been shown to help older adults shed fat from their midsection. A study published in the *Annals of Internal Medicine* compared tai chi with strength training and aerobic exercises. Individuals who practiced tai chi for 12 weeks lost as much weight around the midsection as those who stuck with a traditional aerobic and strength training regime. An additional benefit, those who practiced tai chi regularly for weeks after we're able to maintain better cholesterol levels (Slu et al., 2021).

- Cardio and aerobics. Try to incorporate at least 20 minutes of cardio or aerobic exercise three days a week. This includes walking, jogging, hiking, swimming, dancing, and sports like tennis.

- Resistance training and strength training. Weight-bearing and muscle-strengthening exercises are crucial for maintaining muscles and bone density. After the age of 30, you begin to lose an average of 1% of your muscle every year. Muscle helps you burn through fat and with less of it you are more likely to gain weight. Weight training helps you build and maintain the essential muscles you need to keep fat from being stored around the midsection during menopause. You should try to do strength training two times a week. You can use dumbbells or use elastic bands for more resistant training. Your body weight can be used for strength training. Push-ups and planks are great examples of exercises you can perform that use only your bodyweight to complete. You should be able to do up to 12 repetitions of any weight training move before your muscles become fatigued.

Strength training should activate specific muscle groups like the legs and glutes, core muscles, lower back, and the shoulders and upper arms. There are many basic moves you can perform that activate these muscle groups, some will trigger more than one.

Getting Started

If it has been a while since you exercised or you tell yourself all the time how much you 'hate' exercising, getting started is going to be a real challenge. Keep in mind, it doesn't matter what type of exercise you should be doing. While strength training and cardio workouts can help you lose weight and maintain better health, if these types of workouts aren't your thing then do not do them. As you will learn, the most important thing about sticking with an exercise routine is finding something you enjoy doing and will look forward to doing. If you wake up and go through your day dreading the thought of having to work out, you will be more tempted to skip it or make excuses not to do it.

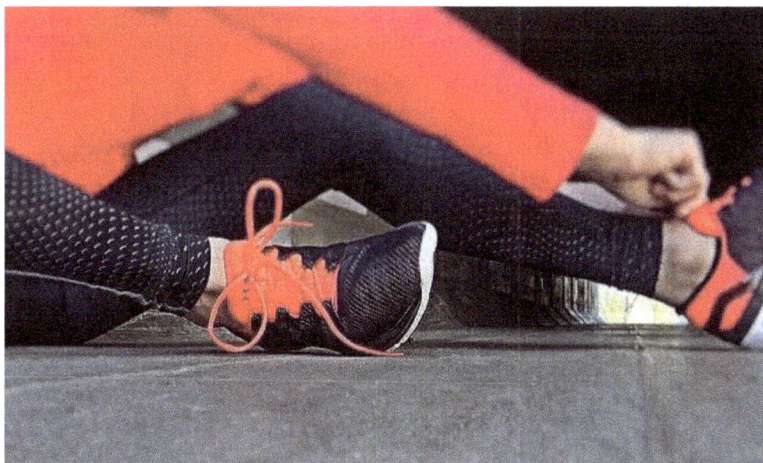

Staying Motivated

As we just mentioned, you want to choose an activity you will enjoy doing. If you hate jogging, do not force yourself to work five days a week. You will only cause more internal struggles and will be more likely to skip your workouts than you take part in them.

The hardest part for most people is just starting their exercise session. You may find yourself putting it off until later and later in the day until you simply have run out of time to do it. This is especially true when you commit to exercising for longer periods of time. Instead of telling yourself, you have to work out for 30 minutes, give yourself permission to just get started and stick with it for 5 or 10 minutes. This is a mental trick, for many once they get started with their workout and commit to the first 10 minutes they are more likely to complete the whole 30 minutes.

Change the way you look at working out. Many people approach working out as a punishment. This stems from the language we use when we talk about working out. When you say things like "I have to work out", you are telling yourself this is something you have no control over is not something you are going to enjoy. A simple adjustment to your phrasing can trick the brain, and body, into thinking your workout is something you are excited about doing. "I get to workout today", is a much more positive way to phrase what you are about to do. This little change can shift your perspective and you will begin to forward to working out instead of dreading it.

Self-motivation is hard to rely on when starting a new habit, like exercising more. Establishing small rewards for yourself can help you stay motivated to get started. While you do not want to always rely on external factors to motivate you to do something you do not want to do, in this case, it can be beneficial to help you set a foundation to make working out a lifelong habit.

In connection with external motivation, what will keep you committed to working out is having a deeply rooted 'why' for working out. Losing weight is a great starting point to establish a why, but this is often just the tip of the iceberg. Why do you want to lose weight? How would losing weight make you feel? What other things will improve once you lose the weight? When you dig a little deeper to fully understand why it is important to you to work so you lose weight there are many potential reasons you can draw upon to get you moving on even the hardest of days.

For example, you may want to lose weight so you can enjoy playing with your kids or grandkids, you want to be able to make memories with them where you are present in what they are doing instead of just sitting and watching from the sidelines. You may want to avoid suffering from serious health risks as you may have witnessed a family member struggle with when you were younger. You may just be tired of waiting for the end to come and instead, want to feel like you are in the best shape of your life because you have many years of life left in you.

Whatever the reason, studies have shown that those who have an emotionally driven reason for doing anything are more likely to succeed in their goals.

Setting Realistic Goals

Setting workout goals will help you track the physical activity you are doing. Keep your first workout goals easy and nearly impossible not to achieve. For example, you might start working out 10 minutes 3 days a week as a beginning goal. From here you can build on these goals. You can either add an extra day of working out for `10 or increase the length of your workout to 15 minutes.

When you set goals like this that are easy to manage and accomplish it will boost your confidence and establish a habit. Once you make working out a habit it turns into something you automatically do. You won't fight with yourself about whether or not you will do it, you will simply put on your workout clothes and get started.

Weekly exercise suggestions:

- One high-intensity session (20 minutes), two moderate sessions (30 minutes each), one strength training session (20 to 30 minutes), one longer aerobic session (45 to 60 minutes), one low-intensity session (30 minutes).

- Two days of high-intensity sessions (20 minutes each), two strength training sessions (30 minutes each), one longer aerobic/cardio session (60 minutes).

- Five low-intensity days (30 minutes each) and one strength training day (30 minutes).

When you are just starting, be flexible with your approach. Do what you know you can commit to, then after two or three weeks re-evaluate your progress. If you feel you can add in more days or want to try a new type of exercise then give yourself permission to do so. Remember, it is about increasing your physical activity a little over time. You can add to the foundation you build as you go. Approaching exercise with a slightly slow yet steady process will better ensure you make working out a daily habit as opposed to a temporary activity you only do to drop some weight.

Keep it simple

Walking is an ideal way to start a regular exercise routine. Walking 10,000 steps a day can help you burn about 400 calories a day. Walking slightly more steps like 11,000 can burn an extra 500 calories a day, which would average to losing 1 pound a week. The faster your walk and resistance, such as walking upstairs or up a hill, can help you burn even more. Setting a step goal for your day and finding ways to walk a little more each day and you will find that losing weight and keeping it off is easier than you think.

Another thing to consider is standing more often during your day. If you have a fairly sedentary lifestyle it is going to be harder to lose weight. If your job has you sitting for most of the day, this will add to your weight gain. Getting up and standing requires the body to exert more effort which means you naturally are burning slightly more calories. If you have a little bit of pacing you can burn even more calories.

One thing to remember as you get started with exercise is to simply find a way to move more and do physical activities that you enjoy. Do not look at exercise as work or something you 'have' to do. Instead, find an activity you really enjoy so it does feel like you are exercising, such as dancing, cycling, swimming, or just playing in the yard with the kids or grandkids. Approach working out as something you 'get' to do and you will notice there is less internal resistance.

Chapter 9:

Additional Lifestyle Changes

After 50, it is not uncommon for women to become more concerned about their overall health. Health conditions become an even bigger concern when you are overweight or worried about your weight. While you cannot completely eliminate the risk for certain conditions, you can make simple adjustments to your daily habits to reduce the risk of things like heart disease and cardiovascular disease. Aside from diet and exercise, there are other lifestyle factors you should evaluate and consider changing during menopause.

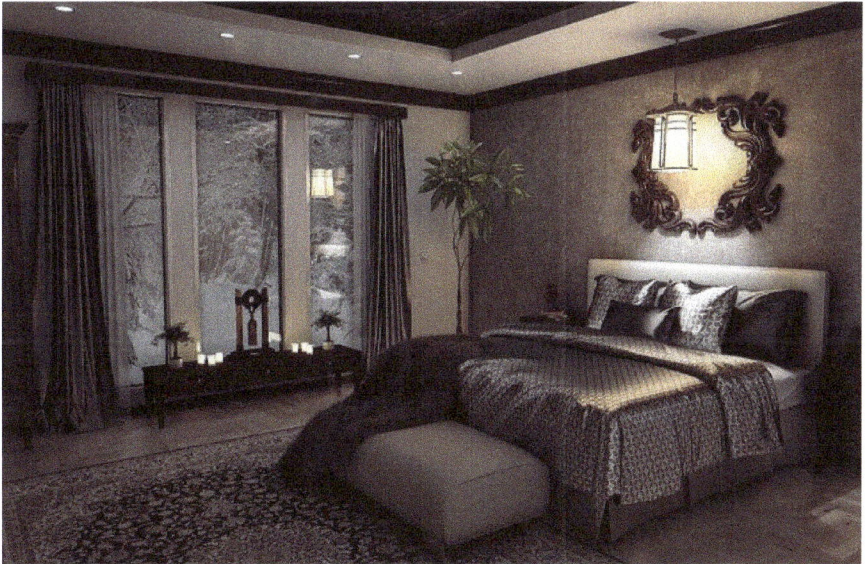

Quality Sleep

Many women struggle to get enough sleep during menopause because of hot flashes, stress, or changes in their hormones. While we all know sleep is important because we need to be well-rested to get through our day, sleep has an impact on much more than just our focus and energy levels.

If you are struggling with your weight, despite eating better and exercising, not getting enough sleep may be the reason for your issues. When we skip out on sleep, even if we get an hour less sleep a night, the body turns on its stress response. We produce more of the hunger hormones that cause us to feel hungry. Additionally, without proper sleep, our body does not produce enough or has a delta in producing our hunger-suppressing hormones so we tend to eat more because we are not getting the signal to stop eating. This leads to us being more hungry throughout the day and eating more than we typically would.

There is also a bidirectional link between sleep and exercise. Individuals who struggle to get enough sleep are less likely to participate in many physical activities the next day while those who wake up well-rested are more likely to work out. In line with this, those who exercise regularly report having little to no sleep struggles while those who do not exercise complain about not being able to fall asleep or frequently wake during the night. Additionally, not getting quality sleep can impact our endurance when we exercise. We might feel like we are exerting a lot of energy and burning plenty of calories when in reality we are not.

Reassess your sleeping environment to make it more inviting, relaxing, and comfortable. Things like light, sound, and temperature can all interrupt sleep. Some tips to help improve your quality of sleep include:

1. Turn down the temperature in your room. Most people will get a better sleep when the temperature in their room is around 67 degrees Fahrenheit. To help combat hot flashes or night sweat you might want to lower the temperature even more to between 60 and 65 degrees.

2. Turn off all electronics at least an hour and a half before bed. This includes your phone. If possible, set your phone across the room or in another room so you are not tempted to check it. Enjoy reading, journaling, or another activity that does not require electronics just before bed.

3. Stick with an evening routine that gets your mind and body ready for sleep. Take a relaxing shower or bath, do a skincare routine, meditate, and prepare what you need for the next few days. Having a consistent routine where you go to bed and get up at the same time every day will make it easier to get the sleep you need to be well-rested the next day.

4. Keep the air circulating in your room. Turn on the ceiling fan to move air around your room which can help you breathe better and will keep you cool. Also, consider getting a dehumidifier for your bedroom which can help reduce night sweats and hot flashes.

Stress Relief and Management

Your weight may be causing you excess stress, and the more you stress about your weight, the more weight you are likely to put on. We also experience stress throughout the day, and many of us deal with much higher levels of stress than others. Your job, finances, relationship, and health can make you stressed. When we experience stress we produce cortisol which puts in motion the body's fight or flight response. When we are in this state the body naturally begins to release blood sugar to give us a boost of energy. On the outside, this may seem like a good thing because this means the body is converting stored energy to usable fuel. But, when we are constantly stressed this can overstimulate the liver leading to insulin resistance and type 2 diabetes.

Minimizing your stress levels and taking time throughout the day to help combat stress can help you keep extra weight off and be better for your overall health. You do not need to spend hours of your day meditating to try to relax your body and mind. Pausing just a few times a day to check in with yourself, your thoughts, and your emotions can help combat fears and anxiety.

Some simple stress reduction practices include:

- meditation
- journaling
- deep breathing exercises
- reading
- practicing gratitude
- getting outside
- add live plants to your work and home environment

If you are unable to find relief from your worry and stress, consider talking to a therapist or counselor. Talking to a professional can help alleviate your worrisome thoughts. You may also find helpful ways to address the behaviors that are being driven by your emotions like emotional eating or lack of motivation.

Therapy

Hormone therapy is commonly prescribed to women going through menopause. Hormone replacement therapy involves taking a low dose of estrogen to help combat hot flashes, night sweats, and mood swings. Estrogen is often taken as a pill but there are also estrogen patches, vaginal rings, spray, and gels.

There are also estrogen and progestin therapies that require you to take a low dose of both estrogen and progesterone. This approach can lower the risk of developing certain cancers like cancer of the endometrium.

Depending on your age, the type of hormone therapy you receive, and health history, hormone therapy comes with some concerning risks. There is a greater chance of suffering from heart disease, breast cancers, having a stroke, and developing blood clots. These are serious conditions that would need to be weighed carefully when considering hormone therapy.

Acupuncture

For women who want an alternative to traditional hormone therapy or those who do not want to pursue hormone therapy, acupuncture can alleviate some menopausal symptoms. Acupuncture has been shown to help women during menopause. Some symptoms it can help relieve include (Bringle, 2021):

- the frequency and severity of hot flashes
- mood swings
- insomnia
- night sweats
- anxiety
- pain
- fatigue

The World Health Organization (WHO) also established a list of conditions acupuncture can help improve or treat which include (Brazier, 2017):

- regulating blood pressure levels
- tension headaches
- migraines
- back and neck pain
- osteoarthritis
- risk of stroke

On top of this, there is a chance that you will feel more energized, less stressed, and experience having an overall better mood after an acupuncture session.

Acupuncture treatment. like all types of treatments does have risk involved and minimal side effects. You may experience bruising, soreness, or bleeding may occur where the needle is inserted. If you have a blood clotting condition or are on blood thinner medication, this type of treatment can be dangerous. Other concerns to be aware of include the risk of infection from unsterile needles. There is also the rare chance that the tip of the needle may break when inserted or removed, which can cause internal damage to the organs. Another rare occurrence that can happen is the needle being inserted too deeply in the chest or upper back areas. Though very few reports of the happening have been reported it can result in the lung being punctured or collapsing.

Keep in mind that these more serious concerns have more to do with the establishment where you are receiving acupuncture treatment. Before deciding to have acupuncture done it is important to research the facility providing the treatment. Find a licensed practitioner that has proper training and experience with acupuncture. You can check to see if the place you are considering has licensed practitioners by visiting the National Certification Commission in Acupuncture and Oriental Medicine (NCCAOM). On the NCCAOM website, you will be able to see which practitioners in your area have been licensed by the board which can give you extra comfort in knowing you are visiting a place that is credible and the staff has the proper training.

A trained professional acupuncturist can also help you identify and address other factors that can contribute to your menopausal symptoms. Many can advise patients on what foods may trigger symptoms, the type of exercise to relieve symptoms, relaxation techniques designed to specifically minimize anxiety and improve mood. Always go with your gut feeling. If you do not feel comfortable with the place or person you will be receiving the treatment from, find another establishment.

Additional Suggestions

Make it a point to visit your doctor regularly to monitor your health. At this age, you should be scheduling regular tests and be aware of the additional check-ups most women neglect. Aside from the most common, mammograms, you want to continue with annual pelvic exams and routine visits to your primary care doctor. Along with these additional tests or check-ups you want to consider are:

- colonoscopy
- thyroid
- blood sugar tests carotid artery ultrasound (to screen for early stages of cardiovascular issues)
- bone mineral density tests
- vitamin B levels and other potential nutrient deficiencies

This is obvious but can't be stressed enough, if you smoke, now is the time to quit. You are probably already aware of all the health risks that come along with smoking but during menopause, these risks increase substantially.

Get enough vitamin D but be careful in the sun. While the sun provides us with essential vitamin D, you might be less tolerable of sun exposure. Burning from too much skin can increase the risk of skin cancer. You will also see more age-related issues with your skin such as wrinkles, sagging around the eyes, and dark spots.

Exercise your brain more. As we age our cognitive function naturally declines. During menopause, women may struggle more with memory loss and difficulty concentrating because of fluctuation hormones. To help combat these problems and to improve brain health you want to incorporate some brain-stimulating activities.

These can include:

- building jigsaw puzzles
- completing crossword puzzles

- playing or learning how to play an instrument
- reading
- playing chess
- knitting or crocheting
- painting, drawing, or sketching

Simply learning something new or picking up a hobby you always want to try can help with cognitive function. When you attempt something you have never done before it triggers the growth of neural connection while also strengthening connections already formed.

Stay hydrated by drinking plenty of water. When you are even the slightest bit dehydrated you can suffer from headaches, fatigue, and are more prone to overeat. Your body consists of mostly water and it is essential for many of the systems in your body to operate properly. If you are the type of person that would much rather reach for a soda, sweet tea, or coffee, try to slowly replace one of these beverages with a glass of water instead. By slowly swapping out these sugar-filled drinks with water you will not only find common symptoms reduced but you will find it easier to manage your weight.

Consider also addressing when you eat, not just how or what you eat. Midnight snacks, mindless eating, and grabbing something quick on the go can all keep you from losing weight. We discussed how mindful and intuitive eating can help combat overeating but another thing to consider as you get older is cutting down on your eating window. Most people follow the idea that they need to eat three big meals and two small snacks throughout the day. But, some studies suggest that menopausal women can help keep extra weight off by sticking to just three meals a day. Breakfast or lunch should be your biggest meals so you fuel the body properly to get through your daily activities. Dinner should be a much smaller meal as the digestive system slows down and may not adequately digest a big meal at the end of the day.

You may always want to consider a type of intermittent fasting eating plan. Simply adhering to a 12-hour window where you fast between your last and first meal can help you burn fat while you sleep. For example, if you make your last meal at 7 p.m., your next meal should be no earlier than 7 a.m.

Chapter 10:

BONUS Recipes

Just because you are going through menopause and watching your weight and health does not mean you need to stick to boring salads and bland meals every day. It can be hard to find the right nutritious recipes that are quick and easy to create week after week, which is why this chapter was included. Here you will find delicious, healthy recipes that you can make a part of your weekly meal plan with ingredients easy to find in your local supermarket.

Breakfast

Goat Cheese and Asparagus Frittata

Servings: 4

Ingredients:
- 12 eggs
- ½ cup cream
- 4 tbsp butter
- 1 leek (white part only, sliced thin)
- 2 bunches of asparagus (trimmed, cut diagonally into 1-inch pieces)
- 2 tbsp dill (chopped)
- ½ cup goat cheese (crumbled)
- whole-wheat toast (for servings)

- 2 cups arugula (for serving)
- 4 tbsp lemon juice (optional)

Directions:

1. Preheat the oven to 400°F (200°C).
2. Add the butter to a cast-iron skillet (or oven-safe frying pan) over medium heat.
3. Add the leeks to the skillet and cook for five minutes or until they begin to soften.
4. Add the asparagus to the skillet and cook for two minutes, or until they are bright green and still crispy.
5. Whisk the eggs, cream, and chopped dill in a large bowl then pour into the cast iron skillet. Stir the eggs, lower the heat and cook for five more minutes. The eggs should be slightly runny still.
6. Turn the heat off and sprinkle the goat cheese over top.
7. Set the skillet in the oven and bake for 15 minutes. The top will be a light golden brown. The center of the eggs should be a little firm but still springy.
8. Cut the frittata into four sections.
9. Serve over the arugula drizzled with fresh lemon juice, and a slice of whole-wheat toast.

Almond Pancakes

Servings: 2 (makes 8)

Ingredients:
- coconut oil (for cooking the pancakes)
- ¾ cup unsweetened almond milk
- 2 eggs
- ⅓ cup oats

- ½ cup almond flour
- 1 tbsp ground flaxseed
- 1 tsp baking powder
- ½ tsp baking soda
- 1 tsp pure vanilla extract
- ½ tsp cinnamon
- ½ tsp sea salt

Directions:

1. Add all the ingredients into a blender, blend for five minutes or until smooth. Set to the side.
2. Place a medium-size frying pan and turn the heat to medium. Heat the pan for five minutes then add a little coconut oil and allow it to melt.
3. Pour a little of the pancake batter into the pan. You want the pancakes to be about three inches across.
4. Cook the pancake for three minutes or until the edges have begun to brown and small bubbles or holes form on the top. Flip and cook for another three minutes or until a nice golden brown.
5. Repeat until all batter is used.
6. Top with fresh blueberries, pure maple syrup, or melted almond butter before servings.
7. Place any leftovers in an airtight container and set them in your fridge for five days.

Overnight Oats

Servings: 1

Ingredients:

- ½ cup oats (steel cut or old fashioned, not instant or quick cook)
- 1 cups almond milk
- 1 tbsp chia seed
- 1 tbsp flax seed (ground)
- 1 tbsp hemp seed
- 1 tbsp honey or pure maple syrup

Directions:

1. Layer all the ingredients into a mason jar, stir, and cover.
2. Refrigerate overnight or at least six hours.
3. Stir in the morning and enjoy!

Additional serving suggestions:

- add a tablespoon of almond butter in the morning.
- top with ¼ cup of Greek yogurt.
- mix in fresh blackberries in the morning.

Breakfast Sweet Potato

Servings: 4

Ingredients:

- 2 tbsp coconut oil (divided)
- 2 sweet potatoes (washed and dried)
- 2 cups Greek yogurt
- 4 tsp cinnamon

- 2 tsp nutmeg
- 1 tsp sea salt

Directions:

1. Preheat the oven to 400°F (200°C) and line a baking sheet with aluminum foil or parchment paper.
2. Use a tablespoon of coconut oil to rub on the potatoes and sprinkle with salt. Place the potatoes on the baking sheet and bake for 45 minutes or until you can easily poke a fork through them.
3. Remove from the oven. Allow the potatoes to cool for five minutes, then cut them in half lengthwise.
4. Use a fork to mash the remaining coconut oil into the sweet potato. Top each half of the sweet potato with a quarter cup of Greek yogurt and sprinkle with cinnamon and nutmeg.
5. You can store the baked potatoes in the refrigerator for up to five days but leave off the toppings.

Egg Muffins

Servings: 6 (makes 12)

Ingredients:
- 1 tbsp olive oil
- 6 eggs
- 2 cups baby spinach (chopped)
- 1 red bell pepper (diced)
- 1 cup mushrooms (chopped)
- 2 garlic cloves (minced)
- 1 tbsp flax seed (ground)

Directions:

1. Preheat the oven to 350°F (175°C) and grease a 12 servings muffin tray or line with muffin cups. Set the tray to the side.
2. In a large frying pan add the oil and place over medium heat. Warm the oil, then add the bell pepper. Cook for five minutes or until tender, then add the mushrooms and garlic. Stir and cook for one more minute. Turn the heat off and set it to the side.
3. Take a large mixing bowl and beat the eggs with the ground flaxseed. Set aside.
4. Take the muffin tray and add the sauteed vegetables to each cup. Take the egg mixture and pour over the vegetables.
5. Bake for 20 minutes or until the eggs have turned a light golden brown.
6. Enjoy!
7. Allow the eggs to cool completely before storing them in the refrigerator, use within five days.

Smoothies

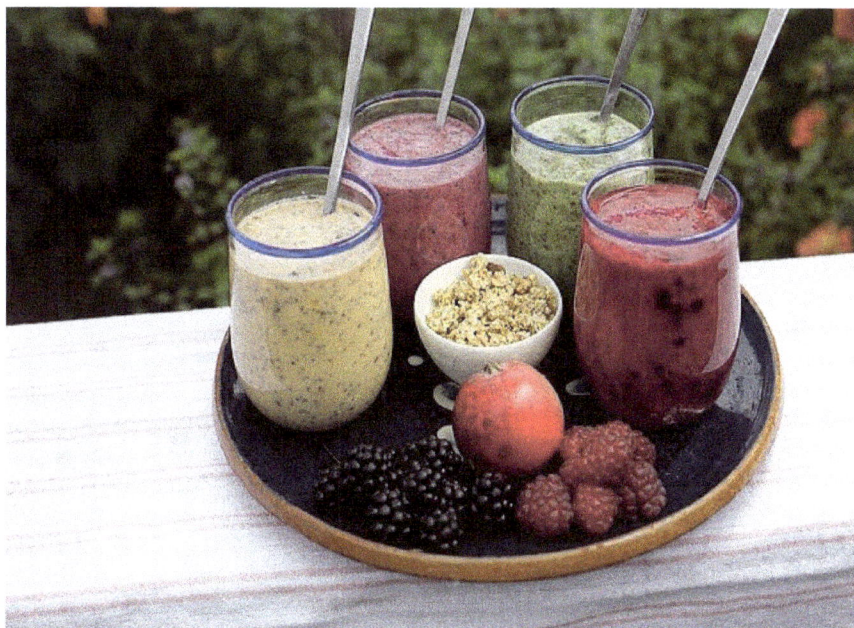

Pineapple Avocado Smoothie

Servings: 2

Ingredients:

- 1 ½ cup orange juice
- 1 tsp lime juice
- 1 ½ cups pineapple (chunks)
- 1 avocado (seed and skin removed)
- 1 tbsp honey
- ½ cup ice

Directions:

1. Add all the ingredients to a blender.
2. Blend for five minutes or until smooth, then enjoy!

Berry Smoothie

Servings: 2

Ingredients:

- 2 cups unsweetened soy milk, almond milk, or water
- ½ cup mixed berries (fresh or frozen)
- 2 tbsp yogurt
- 1 tsp tahini
- ice (if using fresh berries instead of frozen)

Directions:

1. Add all the ingredients to a blender.
2. Blend for five minutes or until smooth, then enjoy!

Banana, Blueberry, Cauliflower Smoothie

Servings: 1

Ingredients:

- 1 cup cauliflower florets (frozen)
- 1 banana (frozen)
- ½ cup blueberries (frozen)
- 4 pitted dates
- 2 tbsp flaxseed
- 2 tbsp hemp seeds
- 1 tbsp raw cacao powder

- 1 tsp matcha powder
- 1 tsp pure vanilla extract

Directions:

1. Add all the ingredients to a blender.
2. Blend for five minutes or until smooth, then enjoy!

Green Smoothie

Servings: 1

Ingredients:

- 1 cup coconut milk
- 1 avocado (seed and peel removed, roughly chopped)
- 1 cucumber (peeled, roughly chopped)
- 2 cups baby spinach
- 1 lime (just the juice)
- 1 tbsp coconut oil
- 1 tsp chia seed
- 1 tsp flaxseed
- ice for a thicker smoothie

Directions:

1. Add all the ingredients to a blender.
2. Blend for five minutes or until smooth, then enjoy!

Mango Banana Smoothie

Servings: 1

Ingredients:
- 1 cup almond milk
- 1 tbsp coconut oil
- 1 cup mangos (frozen or fresh)
- 1 banana
- 1 tbsp lime juice
- 1 tbsp chia seed
- 1 tbsp flaxseed
- 1 tbsp honey

Directions:
1. Add all the ingredients to a blender.
2. Blend for five minutes or until smooth, then enjoy!

Lunch

Eggplant and Broccoli Lemongrass Curry with Tofu

Servings: 4

Ingredients:
- 2 tbsp. coconut oil
- 1 cup vegetable stock
- ½ pound or 10 ounces of firm tofu (cubed)
- 2 apples (diced)
- 4 garlic cloves (chopped fine)

- 1-inch piece ginger (chopped fine)
- 2 stalks of lemongrass (crushed, chopped fine)
- 1 eggplant (cut into wedges)
- 3 cups broccoli (florets)
- 2 tsp. turmeric (ground)
- 1 tsp. mustard seed (ground)
- ½ tsp. chili flakes
- 1 tbsp. apples cider vinegar
- 1 14-ounce can coconut milk
- 1 can chickpeas (rinsed, drained)
- 1 tsp. Himalayan salt
- fresh basil (optional)

Directions:

1. First, press the tofu to release excess water, then set aside.
2. Next place a large stockpot on the stove over medium-high heat. Add the oil and allow it to melt, then add the garlic. Saute for one minute, then add the ginger, lemongrass, turmeric, mustard seed, and chili flakes. Lower the heat to medium, continue to cook the spices for one minute, stirring occasionally.
3. Add the eggplant and apples to the pot. Fry for about five minutes.
4. Pour in the vegetable stock and apple cider vinegar. Stir, cover, and cook for 20 minutes.
5. Remove the lid, pour in the coconut milk, and stir. Add the broccoli, chickpeas, and tofu. Simmer for 10 minutes.
6. Stir in the salt and serve hot.
7. Keep the leftovers in an airtight container for no more than five days.

Avocado and Cucumber Salad with Fresh Herbs and Tahini Dressing

Sevings: 4

Ingredients:

- 1 fresh bunch of coriander
- 1 fresh bunch of purple basil
- 1 avocado
- 1 cup cherry tomatoes (halved)
- 2 cucumbers (small, sliced thin)
- ¼ cup sunflower seeds

For Dressing:

- 3 tbsp tahini
- 2 tbsp tamari
- ¼ teaspoon chili flakes
- ¼ cup warm water (to thin the dressing)

Directions:

1. In a small bowl whisk all dressing ingredients, set to the side.
2. Next, take a large mixing bowl and mix all the remaining ingredients and toss.
3. Divide the salad into four equal portions, drizzle the tahini dressing over top and enjoy.
4. Store the salad and dressing in separate containers. The salad will stay fresh for up to five days, the dressing will be good for up to seven days.

Spinach Salad with Walnuts and Figs

Servings: 4

Ingredients:

- 2 tbsp walnut oil (cold-pressed)
- 2 tbsp balsamic vinegar
- 2 cups baby spinach
- ½ red onion (sliced thin)
- 8 dried figs (sliced)
- ¼ cup black cherries (halved, optional)
- 2 tbsp walnuts (chopped)
- ½ tsp honey
- ¼ tsp sea salt
- ¼ tsp black pepper

Directions:

1. Thoroughly mix the walnut oil, balsamic vinegar, honey, salt, and black pepper in a small mixing bowl. Set aside.
2. Place the spinach, onions, figs, cherries, and walnuts in a large salad bowl and toss.
3. Drizzle the walnut oil dressing over the salad, toss to coat everything evenly, then enjoy!
4. Keep any leftovers in your fridge for up to three days.

Tomato Soup

Servings: 4

Ingredients:

- 2tbsp extra virgin coconut oil
- 1 cup water

- 2 cups cherry tomatoes
- 2 tbsp lemongrass (trimmed, chopped fine)
- 2 tsp fresh ginger (minced)
- 1 tsp fresh basil leaves (sliced thin)
- 1 tsp sea salt

Directions:

1. Place the coconut oil, tomatoes, lemongrass, ginger, and salt into a blender. Blend until smooth, then transfer to a medium-size pot.
2. Set the pot on the stove over medium heat.
3. Allow the soup to become hot.
4. Serve with the fresh basil leaves over top.
5. The soup can be stored in the fridge for up to three days.

Steamed Bok Choy

Servings: 4

Ingredients:

- ¼ teaspoon organic sesame oil
- 1 tsp water
- 1 tbsp soy sauce
- 2 bunches bok choy (ends trimmed, cut to 1-inch pieces)
- 2 garlic cloves (minced)
- 1 tsp ginger (grated)
- ¼ teaspoon black pepper

Directions:

1. Place the bok choy, garlic, and ginger into a steamer basket. Place the basket into a pot with boiling water, be sure the basket is not touching the water. Cover and steam for 30

second or until the leaves of the bok choy have softened but the stem is still firm.

2. Transfer the bok choy from the steamer basket to a serving platter.
3. In a small bowl, whisk the sesame oil, soy sauce, black pepper, and water. Pour mixture over the bok choy and enjoy!
4. Leftovers can be kept for up to three days in your fridge.

Servings Suggestions:

- Serve alongside baked fish, roasted chicken, or grilled meat.
- Serve over a large spinach salad.
- Serve with brown rice or quinoa.
- Seve over shredded cabbage, carrots, cucumber, and radish.

Dinner

Marinated Pork with Pawpaw and Basil Salsa

Servings: 4

Ingredients:
- 2 tablespoon olive oil
- 1 teaspoon red wine vinegar
- 4 x quarter-pound pork medallions (fat trimmed)
- 1 onion (chopped fine)
- 1 papaw or green mango (peeled, seeds removed, chopped)
- 1 teaspoon lemon rind (grated)
- 2 teaspoon lemon juice
- ½ cup basil leaves (shredded)

- 1 teaspoon smoked paprika
- 1 ½ teaspoon sea salt (divided)

Directions:

1. Rub each of the pork medallions with the lemon rind, paprika, and 1 teaspoon of salt. Place the pork in an airtight container and set it in the fridge to marinate for at least two hours.
2. After the pork has marinated, place a grill pan on the stove. Turn the heat to medium so the pan becomes hot. Place the pork on the pan. Cook for three minutes on each side.
3. Place the pork on a plate and cover with aluminum foil. Let the pork rest for five minutes.
4. As the pork rests, prepare the salsa. Place the lemon juice, olive oil, red wine vinegar, onion, papaya, basil leaves, and ½ teaspoon of salt. Toss to combine.
5. Serve the pork with the salsa over top.
6. Keep any leftovers in your fridge for up to five days.

Barley and Coriander Pesto

Servings: 4

Ingredients:

- 1 ½ cups water
- ½ cup vegetable stock
- ½ cup pearl barley
- 8 ozs. whole-wheat spaghetti
- 1 scallion (diced)
- 1 cup cherry tomatoes (halved)
- ¼ cup Parmesan cheese
- 1 bunch fresh coriander
- a handful of fresh arugula

- ¼ teaspoon sea salt
- ¼ teaspoon black pepper

Directions:

1. Place a saucepan on the stove with the water in it and bring to a boil over medium heat. Add the barley, stir, cover, and simmer for 30 minutes.
2. As the barley simmers, cook the pasta according to package instructions. Drain then set in a large mixing bowl.
3. As the pasta cooks, place the coriander, scallions, and half the tomatoes into a food processor. Pulse a few times, then pour in the vegetable stock and parmesan cheese. Blend until smooth, then pour over the pasta.
4. Add the barley, the rest of the tomatoes, arugula, salt, and black pepper. Toss until everything is nicely combined.
5. The leftovers can be stored for up to five days in your fridge.

*For extra protein, top the pasta with hard-boiled eggs, roasted chicken, or poached salmon.

Poach Salmon and Potatoes with Watercress Sauce

Servings: 4

Ingredients:
- 4 tbsp butter (unsalted)
- 1 ½ cups white wine
- 2 lbs skinless salmon filet
- 2 lbs baby potatoes (peeled)
- 2 carrots (chopped)
- 2 stalks of celery (chopped)
- 1 onion (sliced)
- 1 fennel bulb (sliced)

- zest of one lemon (in long pieces not grated)
- 2 flat-leaf parsley stalks
- 2 tbsp parsley leaves (chopped)
- 1 tsp whole black peppercorns

For Sauce:
- 1 cup extra virgin olive oil
- 3 egg yolks
- ½ tsp lemon zest
- 1 tbsp lemon juice
- 1 tbsp Dijon mustard
- ½ cup watercress (chopped)

Directions:
1. Fill a large stock pot with about 10 cups of water. Add the carrots, celery, fennel bulk, parsley stalks, lemon zest, and whole peppercorns. Cover and simmer over medium heat for 30 minutes.
2. Use cheesecloth or muslin to strain the liquid into a deep dish pan. The dish should be big enough to fit the salmon filet in and can be used on the stove. Discard the solids from the liquid.
3. Place the dish on the stove over medium-low heat. Place the salmon in the dish and poach for 10 minutes. Turn off the heat, cover the dish with aluminum foil and let it sit for 20 minutes.
4. As the salmon sits, make the sauce. Add the egg yolks, Dijon mustard, lemon zest, and lemon juice to a food processor. Blitz until combined, then slowly add in the oil until the sauce begins to thicken. Add the watercress, then blend for five minutes or until smooth. The sauce will have the same consistency as mayonnaise. If the sauce is too thick add warm water a tablespoon at a time until desired consistency. Set the sauce in the refrigerator until ready to use.

5. Next, place the small potatoes into a large pot and cover the potatoes with water. Turn the heat to medium, cover, and cook the potatoes for 10 minutes or until they are tender. Strain the water then place the potatoes in a large mixing bowl and toss with the butter and chopped parsley leaves.
6. Remove the salmon from the poaching dish and chopped into pieces.
7. Place some of the potatoes on a plate, top with the poached salmon, and drizzle the sauce over top.
8. The leftovers can be kept in the refrigerator for up to three days.

Cauliflower Mac and Cheese

Servings: 6

Ingredients:
- 8 oz lentil pasta
- 1 tbsp olive oil
- ½ cup vegetable stock
- 1 cup cauliflower florets
- 1 yellow onion (diced)
- 2 garlic cloves (minced)
- 2 tsp thyme (minced)
- ¼ tsp nutmeg
- ¼ cup plus 3 tbsp nutritional yeast
- 1 cup cheddar cheese (shredded)
- 1 tsp Dijon mustard
- ¼ tsp sea salt
- ¼ tsp black pepper
- ¼ cup Panko breadcrumbs

Directions:

1. Preheat the oven to 350°F (175°C).
2. Bring a large pot of water to a boil. Add the cauliflower florets to the pot, cover, and cook for about five minutes or until tender. Strain and set aside.
3. In a frying pan cook the onions, garlic, and thyme for five minutes or medium heat, or until the onions and garlic have started to turn a golden brown. Add the Dijon mustard and nutmeg and cook for another minute.
4. Transfer the onion mixture to a blender and add the cauliflower florets and ¾ cup nutritional yeast. Pour in the stock and blend until you have a thick creamy sauce. Set aside.
5. Next, cook the lentil pasta according to the package direction. Strain and transfer to a large mixing bowl.
6. Pour the sauce over the pasta, use a rubber spoon to stir, and coat everything evenly. Transfer the pasta to an 8x10-inch baking dish. Sprinkle the cheddar cheese, Panko bread crumbs, and the remaining three tablespoons of nutritional yeast over top.
7. Bake for 30 minutes or until the top has turned a light golden brown and is beginning to bubble.
8. Keep leftovers in an airtight container in your fridge for no more than three days.

Mushroom Burgers

Servings: 4

Ingredients:

- 1 tbsp coconut oil
- 2 eggs (lightly beaten)
- 2 cups mushrooms (chopped fine)

- ½ cup onion (chopped fine)
- ½ cup panko bread crumbs
- ¼ cup chickpea flour, almond flour, or buckwheat flour
- ½ cup shredded cheddar cheese
- ¼ tsp thyme (dried)
- ½ tsp salt
- ½ tsp black pepper
- 4 whole-wheat buns
- lettuce, tomato, and avocado (optional for topping)

Directions:

1. In a large mixing bowl combine the mushrooms, eggs, panko bread crumbs, cheese, onion, flour, thyme, salt, and pepper. Use your hands or a rubber spatula to stir everything.
2. Divide the mixture into four equal portions and shape it into thick burger patties. Set to the side.
3. Set a large skillet on the stove. Turn the heat to medium, then add the coconut oil and allow the oil to melt.
4. Place the burgers in the hot skillet. Cook for four minutes on each side or until they are a crispy golden brown.
5. Remove from the skillet and place each patty on a whole wheat pun. Top with your favorite burger toppings.
6. Leftovers can be kept in the refrigerator for five days.

Snacks

Kale Chips

Servings: 10

Ingredients:

- 8 cups kale leaves (firmly packed, stalks removed)
- 1 cup cashews (soaked in water for three hours, drained, rinsed)
- 2 tbsp water (more if needed)
- 3 tbsp lemon juice
- 8 garlic cloves (chopped)
- 4 tsp garlic powder
- 1 tbsp agave nectar (optional)
- 1 tsp sea salt

Directions:

1. Preheat your oven to 350°F (175°C).
2. Add the soaked cashews, lemon juice, garlic cloves, agave nectar, and sea salt to a food processor. Blitz several times then pour in the water and blend until smooth. The mixture should be similar in consistency to hummus, if necessary add more water one tablespoon at a time.
3. Place the kale leaves into a large mixing bowl and spoon half the cashew mixture over top. Message the mixture into the leaves, then add the remaining cashew mixture and message the leaves again.
4. Spread the kale onto a baking sheet lined with parchment paper, then sprinkle the garlic powder over top.

5. Bake the kale for 15 minutes, remove it from the oven, and carefully flip the leaves. Return to the oven and bake for 15 more minutes. The leaves should be nice and crispy.
6. Store the kale chips in an airtight container on your countertop for three days.

Orange Creamsicle Chia Pudding

Servings: 2

Ingredients:
- 1 cup almond milk
- 1 tsp orange zest
- ¼ tsp pure vanilla extract
- 3 tbsp chia seeds
- honey (optional, to drizzle on top)
- 4 tbsp coconut cream

Directions:
1. Pour the almond milk into a medium-sized mixing bowl then add the orange zest, vanilla, and chia seeds. Whisk and let it sit for 15 minutes.
2. Whisk the mixture again to break up any clumps of seeds. Cover and place in your refrigerator. Chill for two hours or until the mixture is a pudding consistency.
3. Stir before serving.
4. To serve, top with two tablespoons of coconut cream and a drizzle of honey.
5. Store the pudding in your fridge for up to five days.

Guacamole

Servings: 8 (makes 2 cups)

Ingredients:

- 3 avocados (pitted and halved)
- ⅓ cup red onion (mixed)
- 1 garlic clove (minced)
- 1 lime (juice)
- 1 tbsp cilantro (chopped)
- ¼ tsp sea salt
- ¼ tsp black pepper

Directions:

1. Remove the flesh from the avocado and place it into a medium-sized mixing bowl. Use a fork to lightly mash the avocado so you have a slightly chunky consistency.
2. Add the red minion, minced garlic, lime juice, and cilantro to the bowl with the avocado. Mix thoroughly.
3. Season with salt and pepper.
4. Cover with plastic wrap and chill until ready to serve. The guacamole will stay fresh for up to three days when stored in the fridge.

Serving Suggestions:

- Top burgers, wraps, or sandwiches for extra flavor.
- Serve with corn tortilla chips.
- Fill mini sweet peppers or serve with raw vegetable sticks.

Hummus

Servings: 20 (2 tablespoons per serving)

Ingredients:
- 3 tbsp extra virgin olive oil (plus more for topping)
- 15-ounce can chickpeas (drained, rinsed)
- 2 garlic cloves
- ½ cup tahini
- ½ tsp baking soda
- ½ tsp cumin
- 2 tbsp lemon juice
- ½ tsp sea salt
- ½ cup cold water
- paprika or za'atar (optional for topping)

Directions:
1. Place the rinsed chickpeas in a clean kitchen towel and roll them to separate the skins. Discard the skin and set the chickpeas aside.
2. Bring a small pot of water to a boil then add the chickpeas and baking soda. Boil for 10 minutes or until the chickpeas have softened. Drain the water, then transfer the chickpeas to a food processor.
3. Add the garlic cloves, tahini, cumin, lemon juice, and salt to the food processor. Blitz until smooth. Pause every once in a while to scrape down the side.
4. Begin to add the water to the food processor ¼ cup at a time. Blend for about 5 minutes, or until everything is nicely incorporated.
5. Continue to add what and blend until the hummus is at your desired consistency.

6. Transfer the hummus to a serving bowl and top with extra virgin olive oil, paprika, or za'atar.
7. Keep the hummus in an airtight container. The hummus will stay fresh for up to three days in the fridge. You can also freeze it for up to three months.
8. Serve with whole-wheat pita. vegetable stick, or top of sandwich, wraps, or salads.

Roasted Almonds

Servings: 8 (makes 2 cups)

Ingredients:
- 2 tsp coconut oil
- 2 cups raw almonds
- 3 tbsp honey
- 2 tbsp sugar
- ½ tsp pure vanilla extract
- ½ tsp cinnamon
- 2 tsp water
- ¼ tsp salt

Directions:
1. Preheat the oven to 350°F (175°C).
2. Line a baking sheet with parchment paper, then spread the almonds onto the baking sheet in a single layer. Bake for 10 minutes or until the almonds have turned a deep brown. Stir halfway through. Remove from the oven and let it cool completely.
3. In a small mixing bowl, stir the cinnamon, sugar, and salt. Set aside.

4. Place a large saucepan on the stove over medium-high heat. Add the water, honey, coconut oil, and pure vanilla extract. Bring to a boil, whisk continually.
5. Add the almond to the saucepan and cook for three minutes. Most of the liquid should have been absorbed. Stir frequently.
6. Add half the cinnamon and sugar mixture to the saucepan. Cook for another two minutes or until the mixture begins to caramelize.
7. Transfer the almond to a mixing bowl and sprinkle over the remaining cinnamon-sugar mixture. Toss to coat everything evenly, then spread the almonds out on parchment paper in a single layer.
8. Allow the almond to cool completely.
9. Store on your countertop in an airtight container for five days.

*You can use this recipe to make roasted walnuts or pecans instead of almonds.

Deserts

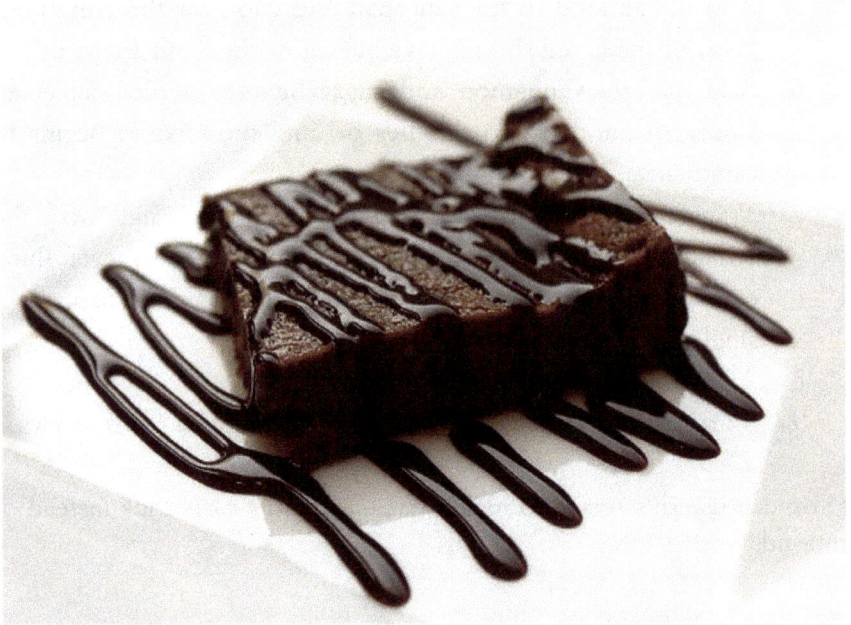

Baked Apple Crisp

Servings: 9

Ingredients:

- 6 honey-crisp apples (peeled, core removed, and sliced thin)
- ⅓ cup pure maple syrup
- 1 tbsp pure vanilla extract
- 1 tsp cinnamon
- ½ tsp nutmeg

For the topping:

- ¼ cup coconut oil (chilled)

- ¼ cup almond flour
- ½ cup old fashioned oats
- ¼ cup dark brown sugar
- ½ cup raw pecans (chopped)
- ¼ tsp cinnamon
- ¼ tsp sea salt

Directions:

1. Preheat your oven to 350°F (175°C) and grease an 8x8-inch baking dish. Set the dish to the side.
2. First, prepare the topping. Stir the flour, oats, brown sugar, pecans, cinnamon, and sea salt into a mixing bowl. It is easiest to use your hands to mix in the chilled coconut oil. You should have a grainy, crumbly mixture. Set the topping in the fridge while you prepare the rest of the dish.
3. Place the sliced apples, maple syrup, vanilla extract, cinnamon, and nutmeg in a large mixing bowl. Stir with a rubber spatula to coat the apples with the rest of the ingredients. Allow the apples to sit for 10 minutes.
4. Take the topping mixture out of the fridge and mix a third of it in with the apples. Transfer the apples to the baking dish and sprinkle the remaining topping mixture over top.
5. Set the baking dish on a baking sheet (in case it bubbles over a bit) and bake for 45 minutes or until the top has turned a golden brown color and is beginning to bubble.
6. Allow the crips to cool for 10 minutes before servings. You can top the crips with whipped coconut cream if you like.
7. Store any remaining crips in your fridge for up to five days. You can assemble the apple crisps and freeze it without baking. Cover the apples with aluminum foil and freeze for up to three months. When you are ready to bake place in the oven for an hour at 350°F.

Black Bean Avocado Brownies

Servings: 12

Ingredients:

- 1 15-ounce can of black beans (drained, rinsed)
- 2 flax eggs (mix two tablespoons of ground flaxseed with six tablespoons of water and let sit for five minutes
- ½ an avocado
- ½ cup and 2 tbsp of dark chocolate chips
- ½ cup dark brown sugar
- ¼ cup pure maple syrup
- ½ cup unsweetened cocoa powder
- ½ tsp baking powder
- ¼ tsp baking soda
- ¼ tsp salt

Directions:

1. Preheat the oven to 350°F (175°C) and grease an 8x8-inch baking dish, then set to the side.
2. Place all ingredients except the dark chocolate chips into a food processor. Blitz until you have a thick smooth mixture. If the mixture is too thick and won't blend, add a little water one teaspoon at a time to help, but do not add too much water, the batter needs to be thick.
3. Fold in 1/3 cup of the dark chocolate chips, then transfer the batter to the baking dish. Sprinkle the remaining chocolate chips over top.
4. Bake in the oven for 30 or until bake all the way through.
5. Let the brownies cool completely, then cut into 12 equal squares.
6. Keep the brownies in an airtight container for no more than five days in your fridge.

Dark Chocolate Chip Cookies

Servings: 12 (makes 24)

Ingredients:

- 6 tbsp coconut oil
- 1 egg
- 4 tbsp Greek yogurt
- 1 zucchini (shredded, squeezed to remove excess water)
- ½ cup coconut sugar
- 4 tbsp honey or pure maple syrup
- 1 tsp pure vanilla extract
- 1 cup whole wheat flour
- ½ cup oats
- ½ tsp cinnamon
- 1 ½ tsp baking powder
- ¼ tsp baking soda
- ½ cup dark chocolate chips
- ½ tsp sea salt

Directions:

1. Preheat the oven to 350°F (175°C) and grease a baking sheet or line with parchment paper. Set to the side.
2. Take a large mixing bowl and add the flour, oat, cinnamon, baking powder, and baking soda, stir, then set aside.
3. In another large bowl use an electric hand mixer (or mix by hand) to beat the coconut oil and coconut sugar, then add the egg, Greek yogurt, honey, and vanilla. Mix until thoroughly incorporated then fold in the shredded zucchini.
4. Take the flour mixture and add one cup at a time to the zucchini mixture. Use a wooden spoon to thoroughly mix everything before adding another cup. Continue until

everything is mixed in one bowl, then fold in the chocolate chips.

5. Next, form the dough into 1-inch size balls and place them on the prepared baking sheet.

6. Bake for 14 minutes or until the cookies have turned an irresistible golden brown. Remove, transfer the cookies to a wire rack, and let them cool completely then enjoy!

7. Keep the cookies in an airtight container on your countertop. They will stay fresh for up to five days.

Cinnamon Raisin Almond Cake

Servings: 16

Ingredients:
- 1 cup olive oil
- 5 eggs
- 1 cup almond milk
- 1 cup soy milk
- 3 cups all-purpose flour
- 2 cups almond flour
- 4 tsp baking soda
- 1 cup almonds (chopped)
- 1 cup raisins
- 2 tsp cinnamon (plus more for sprinkling over top)
- 1 tsp cloves (ground)
- honey (to drizzle over top)

Directions:
1. Preheat the oven to 350°F (175°C) and grease a bundt pan or a 9-inch cake pan. Set to the side.

2. Mix both the flours and baking soda in a mixing bowl. Set aside.

3. Use an electric mixer to beat the olive oil and sugar. Mix for 10 minutes then add the eggs one at a time and mix for 5 minutes. Add both kinds of milk, raisins, almonds, cinnamon, and ground cloves. Mix until nicely combined.

4. Slowly add the flour mixture to the milk and egg mixture. Use a rubber spatula to thoroughly combine everything. Transfer the batter into the bundt pan and bake for 1 hour or until cooked all the way through, use a toothpick to test doneness.

5. Allow it to cool slightly before removing it from the bundt pan. Drizzle honey over top and sprinkle with cinnamon.

6. Keep in the refrigerator for seven days, or individually wrap each serving in parchment paper and plastic wrap to store in the freezer for three months.

Lemon Olive Oil Cake with Blueberry Compote

Servings: 16

Ingredients:

- 1 cup olive oil
- 1 cup Greek yogurt
- 5 egg yolks
- 2 cups all-purpose flour
- 1 cup almond flour
- 1 cup brown sugar
- 2 tsp lemon zest

For the Blueberry Compote

- ½ cup water
- 2 cups blueberries

- 2 strips of lemon zest
- ½ lemon (juice only)
- ½ cup pure maple syrup
- ¼ tsp sea salt

Directions:

1. Preheat the oven to 350°F (175°C) and grease a 9x9-inch baking pan. Set aside.
2. Combine the all-purpose flour and almond flour with the baking powder and lemon zest in a mixing bowl. Stir with a rubber spatula and set to the side.
3. In another larger mixing bowl, beat the olive oil, yogurt, and brown sugar using an electric mixer. Beat for 10 minutes then add one egg yolk at a time and mix until smooth. Slowly add in the flour mixture and beat until everything is thoroughly combined. Transfer the mixture to the grease baking pan.
4. Bake for one hour or until cooked all the way through.
5. As the cake bakes, prepare the blueberry compote. Add the water, blueberries, maple syrup, and lemon zest to a saucepan. Bring to a boil over medium heat, then lower the heat and allow everything to simmer for 10 minutes. For a thicker sauce allow the mixture to simmer for 10 minutes longer. Turn the heat off, and remove the lemon peels. Stir in the lemon juice and sea salt, then allow the mixture to cool completely.
6. When the cake is done baking, allow it to cool before removing it from the pan. Cut into 16 equal pieces and serve each slice with a scoop of blueberry compote over top.

Conclusion

This book has provided you with an in-depth understanding of what to expect leading up to and through menopause. With this understanding, you can begin to take action to feel your best. While you now have a better understanding of what your body is going through, it is also important that you speak to your doctor as well. Talk to your doctor before you begin your new healthy habits. This will allow you to discuss any concerns you may have about changing your diet or increasing physical activity. They may also provide you with additional tips or strategies to manage menopause symptoms and control your weight.

As you have learned, what you eat can help you embrace and enjoy your menopause years or it can add to the discomfort and negative effects. You can either continue to ignore how food affects you and feel sluggish and like the best days of your life have gone by. Or... Wouldn't you rather feel at your best and age like fine wine?

By making simple changes to what you heat, how you eat, and when you eat you will experience a shift in your energy. If you then add in a little more physical activity, you will start to feel like you are in the best shape of your life.

While this book has covered the core factors to weight gain during menopause—diet and exercise—it has also brought to light additional lifestyle choices that can be holding you back. When you combine all the tips and suggestions provided throughout this book, there is no reason why you should dread menopause. However, it is up to you to take action with this new information. All these changes do not need to be made all at once. Simply choose one thing to start with and build from there. If you feel your diet is fairly taken care of but you need to get moving, start by walking just 10 minutes a day. If there are things in your diet you know you need to change, start with one thing at a time, swap out your soda for water, grab a piece of fruit to snack on, or fill half your plate with vegetables and eat those first. These small changes will compound and add up to big changes!

If you are looking for additional dieting plan options that will help you lose weight check out *Top 20 Diets for Weight Loss: A Guide to the Top-Ranked Diets Plus a 7-Day Meal Plan to Get Started for a Healthier, More Energized, and Slimmer You.* This book outlines the best diets that will help you lose weight based on your personal goals and other health conditions. You will learn which low-carb diet is best for you (Atkin's, Keto, Paleo), the best diet to lose weight and improve cognitive function, what diet can help reduce inflammation, and whether you should go gluten-free. *Top 20 Diets for Weight Loss* cover the diets mentioned in this book but go more in-depth in how to get started, benefits, and obstacles you may face when getting started.

Menopause won't last forever. Just as suddenly as it began it will end. You will move on to a new and exciting phase in your life! Why not start this new phase at your healthiest? I wish you luck as you start this new journey and hope that with the information in this book you love the journey!

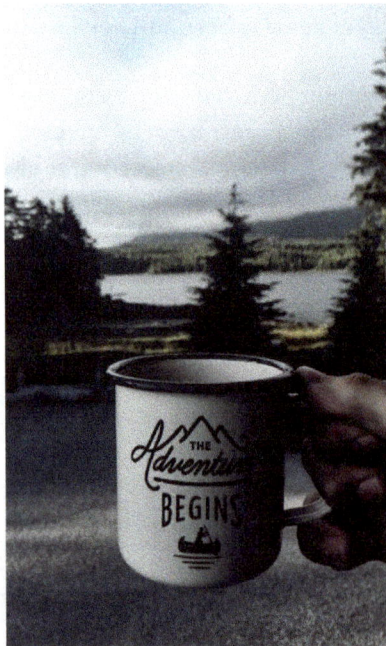

References

3 diet changes women over 50 should make right now. (n.d.). Mayo Clinic. https://www.mayoclinic.org/healthy-lifestyle/nutrition-and-healthy-eating/in-depth/3-diet-changes-women-over-50-should-make-right-now/art-20457589#:~:text=For%20women%20over%2050%2C%20experts

Acosta Scott, J. (2019, April 18). *6 Foods to avoid during menopause.* Everyday Health. https://www.everydayhealth.com/hs/menopause-resource-center/foods-to-avoid/

Alkon, C. (2018, December 31). *Fitness at 40 and beyond: What to know about midlife exercise needs.* Everyday Health. https://www.everydayhealth.com/menopause/know-about-midlife-exercise-needs/

Australian Menopause Centre Staff. (n.d.). *Recipes.* Australian Menopause Centre. Retrieved February 11, 2022, from https://www.menopausecentre.com.au/information-centre/articles/category/recipes/

Bakekal, N. (n.d.). *Plant-based recipes.* Dr. Nitu Bajekal Women's Health Expert. https://nitubajekal.com/resources/recipes/

Barnard, N. D., Kahleova, H., Holtz, D. N., Del Aguila, F., Neola, M., Crosby, L. M., & Holubkov, R. (2021). The Women's Study for the Alleviation of Vasomotor Symptoms (WAVS): a randomized, controlled trial of a plant-based diet and whole soybeans for postmenopausal women. *Menopause: The Journal of the North American Menopause Society*, *28*(10), 1150–1156. https://doi.org/10.1097/GME.0000000000001812

Barnard, N. D., Levin, S. M., & Yokoyama, Y. (2015). A Systematic Review and Meta-Analysis of Changes in Body Weight in Clinical Trials of Vegetarian Diets. *Journal of the Academy of Nutrition and Dietetics*, *115*(6), 954–969. https://doi.org/10.1016/j.jand.2014.11.016

Beezhold, B., Radnitz, C., McGrath, R. E., & Feldman, A. (2018). Vegans report less bothersome vasomotor and physical menopausal symptoms than omnivores. *Maturitas*, *112*, 12–17. https://doi.org/10.1016/j.maturitas.2018.03.009

Brazier, Y. (2017, December 21). *How does acupuncture work?* Medical News Today. https://www.medicalnewstoday.com/articles/156488#how_does_it_work

Breus, M. J. (2010, February 8). *Eating your way to a good night's sleep.* Psychology Today. https://www.psychologytoday.com/us/blog/sleep-newzzz/201002/eating-your-way-good-night-s-sleep#:~:text=Legumes%3A%20Beans%20and%20other%20legumes

Bringle, J. (2021, May 26). *Acupuncture for menopause: How this alternative therapy brought me relief.* Healthline. https://www.healthline.com/health/menopause/acupuncture-for-menopause-how-this-alternative-therapy-brought-me-relief

DASH diet: What is it, meal plans and recipes. (2021, June 18). Cleveland Clinic. https://health.clevelandclinic.org/dash-diet-what-is-it-meal-plans-and-recipes/

Diet type: Recipes. (n.d.). Ambitious Kitchen. https://www.ambitiouskitchen.com/diet/

Elliott, B. (2020, August 27). *The 9 best foods to eat before bed.* Healthline Media. https://www.healthline.com/nutrition/9-foods-to-help-you-sleep

Garrard, C. (2021, July 13). *12 ways to beat menopausal belly fat.* Everyday Health. https://www.everydayhealth.com/menopause-pictures/ways-to-beat-menopausal-belly-fat.aspx

Healthnews International. (2017, September 4). *Amino acids and what they do for menopause.* Newsmaker. https://www.newsmaker.com.au/news/336654/amino-acids-and-what-they-do-for-menopause#.YhId49_MJPZ

Herber-Gast, G.-C. M., & Mishra, G. D. (2013). Fruit, Mediterranean-style, and high-fat and -sugar diets are associated with the risk of night sweats and hot flushes in midlife: results from a prospective cohort study. *The American Journal of Clinical Nutrition, 97*(5), 1092–1099. https://doi.org/10.3945/ajcn.112.049965

Huizen, J. (2019, January 25). *Which foods can help you sleep?* Medical News Today. https://www.medicalnewstoday.com/articles/324295#summary

Link, R., & Northrop, A. (2020, August 28). *Can the keto diet help with menopause?* Healthline. https://www.healthline.com/nutrition/keto-and-menopause#bottom-line

Low-carb and keto recipe collections. (n.d.). Diet Doctor. https://www.dietdoctor.com/low-carb/recipes/collections

Mayo Clinic Staff. (2020, June 9). *Hormone therapy: Is it right for you?* Mayo Clinic. https://www.mayoclinic.org/diseases-conditions/menopause/in-depth/hormone-therapy/art-20046372#:~:text=Hormone%20replacement%20therapy%20is%20medication

Mediterranean diet is linked to higher muscle mass, bone density after menopause. (2018, March 19). Endocrine Society. https://www.endocrine.org/news-and-advocacy/newsroom/2018/mediterranean-diet-is-linked-to-higher-muscle-mass-bone-density-after-menopause

Modern and traditional Mediterranean diet recipes. (n.d.). Mediterranean Living. https://www.mediterraneanliving.com/mediterranean-diet-recipes/

Mushroom burgers. (n.d.). Taste of Home. https://www.tasteofhome.com/recipes/mushroom-burgers/

Ready-Webster, J. (n.d.). *Top recipes with menopause-friendly foods.* Stella. https://www.onstella.com/the-latest/your-body/top-recipes-with-menopause-friendly-foods/

Sacks, F. M., Moore, T. J., Appel, L. J., Obarzanek, E., Cutler, J. A., Vollmer, W. M., Vogt, T. M., Karanja, N., Svetkey, L. P., Lin, P.-H., Bray, G. A., & Windhauser, M. M. (1999). A dietary approach to prevent hypertension: A review of the dietary approaches to stop hypertension (DASH) study. *Clinical Cardiology,* *22*(S3), 6–10. https://doi.org/10.1002/clc.4960221503

Salty foods: How sodium affects your weight. (n.d.). Creekside Family Practice. https://www.creeksidefamilypractice.com/blog/salty-foods-how-sodium-affects-your-weight#:~:text=To%20add%20to%20the%20problem

Shepherd, C. (n.d.). *10 smoothie recipes for menopause.* YourNewLifePlan. https://www.yournewlifeplan.com/10-smoothie-recipes-menopause

Siu, P. M., Yu, A. P., Chin, E. C., Yu, D. S., Hui, S. S., Woo, J., Fong, D. Y., Wei, G. X., & Irwin, M. R. (2021). Effects of Tai Chi or Conventional Exercise on Central Obesity in Middle-Aged and Older Adults. *Annals of Internal Medicine.* https://doi.org/10.7326/m20-7014

Spritzler, F. (2020, April 3). *Why some women gain weight around menopause.* Healthline Media.

https://www.healthline.com/nutrition/menopause-weight-gain#hormones-and-metabolism

The Original Intuitive Eating Pros. (n.d.). *10 Principles of intuitive eating*. Intuitive Eating. https://www.intuitiveeating.org/10-principles-of-intuitive-eating/

Top 10 foods to restore hormone balance. (n.d.). Nutrition 4 Change. https://nutrition4change.com/articles/top-10-foods-to-restore-hormone-balance/

Vegan main dishes. (n.d.). Veggies Don't Bite. https://www.veggiesdontbite.com/category/main-dish/

Vegan Recipes. (n.d.). Yum Vegan Blog. https://yumveganlunchideas.com/

Wal, J. V., Gupta, A., Khosla, P., & Dhurandhar, N. V. (2008). Egg breakfast enhances weight loss. *International Journal of Obesity*, *32*(10), 1545–1551. https://doi.org/10.1038/ijo.2008.130

West, H. (2018, October 17). *The complete beginner's guide to the DASH diet*. Healthline; Healthline Media. https://www.healthline.com/nutrition/dash-diet#what-it-is

Whiteman, H. (2018, February 26). *The diet that could reduce the risk of depression*. Medical News Today. https://www.medicalnewstoday.com/articles/321010

Image References

Akyurt, E. (2021, January 11). [*healthy, fresh, raw vegetables and fruit*] {digital image}. Retrieved from Unsplash. https://unsplash.com/photos/Y5n8mCpvlZU

Bazzocco, M. (2018, November 23). [*Gut Health bowl*] {digital image} Retrieved from Unsplash. https://unsplash.com/photos/qKbHvzXb85A

Boesen, N. (2018, March 13). [*fruit dessert*] {digital image} Retrieved from Pixabay. https://pixabay.com/photos/fruit-dessert-food-drinking-snack-3222313/

Buissinne, S. (2015, January 10). [*physiotherapy*] {digital image}. Retrieved from Pixabay. https://pixabay.com/photos/physiotherapy-weight-training-595529/

Cattalin. (2014, November 7). [*salmon*] {digital image}. Retrieved from Pixabay. https://pixabay.com/photos/salmon-fish-seafood-veggies-salad-518032/

Chaturvedula, S. (2021, January 14). [*casual breakfast setup*] {digital image} Retrieved from Unsplash. https://unsplash.com/photos/sHu3yTbaJvU

Kamatsos, Y. (2014, December 2). [*brownie*] {digital image} Retrieved from Pixabay. https://pixabay.com/photos/brownie-dessert-cake-sweet-548591/

McCutcheon, K. (2018, June 11). [*breakfast in Neükollin*] {digital image}. Retrieved from Unsplash. https://unsplash.com/photos/8qFPuK-tBuY

Raic, V. (2014, July 30). [*scale and tape*] {digital image}. Retrieved from Pixabay. https://pixabay.com/photos/scale-diet-fat-health-tape-weight-403585/

Ramoskaite, D. (2019, October 4). [*strawberry, spinach, and feta salad*] {digital image}. Retrieved from Unsplash. https://unsplash.com/photos/xX9SmqQCbFY

Regan-Asante, s. (2020, November 24). [*steak and vegetables plate*] {digital image}. Retrieved from Unsplash. https://unsplash.com/photos/e3AA8nJMwTI

Rita E. (2017, March 23) [*asparagus*] {digital image}. Retrieved from Pixabay. https://pixabay.com/photos/asparagus-steak-veal-steak-veal-2169313/

Silviarita (2017, May 12). [*fresh fruit bowls*] {digital image}. Retrieved from Pixabay. https://pixabay.com/photos/fresh-fruits-bowls-fruit-bowls-2305192/

Silviarita (2017, September 16). [*salad*] {digital image}. Retrieved from Pixabay. https://pixabay.com/photos/salad-fruit-berry-healthy-vitamins-2756467/

Sleeper, M. (2016, August 16). [*the adventure begins*] {digital image} Retrieved from Unsplash. https://unsplash.com/photos/Spdu7YT1O00

Socha, A. (2018, October 29). [*interior design*] {digital image} Retrieved from Pixabay. https://pixabay.com/photos/bedroom-interior-design-style-3778695/

Svitlana. (2020, July 13). [*tea cup*] {digital image} Retrieved from Unsplash. https://unsplash.com/photos/eXw6CPGWwcg

Total Shape (2020, November 4). [*weight loss*] {digital image} Retrieved from Unsplash. https://unsplash.com/photos/p7nwvfcjk-I

Wellington, J. (2015, January 8). [*woman*] {digital image} Retrieved from Pixabay. https://pixabay.com/photos/woman-girl-freedom-happy-sun-591576/

Wokanda Pix (2016, April 26). [*fitness*] {digital image} Retrieved from Pixabay. https://pixabay.com/photos/fitness-workout-sport-exercise-1348867/

www.ingramcontent.com/pod-product-compliance
Lightning Source LLC
Chambersburg PA
CBHW060043030426

42334CB00019B/2461